Preconception Plain & Simple

A Deliciously Smart and Sexy Guide in Preparing for Pregnancy!

Audrey Couto McClelland and Sharon K. Couto

Pinks & Blues Publishing

BRISTOL, RHODE ISLAND | NEW YORK, NEW YORK

Pinks & Blues Publishing, a division of Whispers Press, LLC
P.O. Box 687, Bristol, RI 02809
www.pinksandblues.com

The information, suggestions, guides, and ideas in this book are neither intended, nor implied, to supersede or substitute the advice or recommendations of trained medical professionals. The authors and the publisher disclaim any liability or responsibility for any use, arising directly or indirectly, of this book. Consult your physician or health-care provider before adopting any suggestions or ideas in this book, as well as about any condition(s), diagnosis(es), or circumstance(s) that may require medical attention.

ISBN 0-975-44260-0 (pbk)

Library of Congress Control Number: 2004106863

Graphic Design: Orange Dot Design | Richard Couto
Cover Illustration: Lyn Fletcher
First printing: September 2004
Printed in the U.S.A. by Barrington Printing, Cranston, RI 02920

For acknowledgments of the use of copyrighted material, see pages 234 - 235.

For Matthew! Oh, Matthew, I could not have written this book without your constant love and support. I love you more than anything in this world. Thank you for believing in this book as much as I do. Thank you for being there for me, either with a suggestion, a new tidbit, or something simply to make me laugh! Ah, yes... and thank you for letting me experiment with everything in this book... on you, and with you! You are not only my husband, but my best friend... and now the father of our son, and our future children! And for William!... the thoughts of conceiving you kept me researching and writing and working with your Grandmother for many wonderful months! Never once did we stop until this book was written... and you were conceived one week later! For you, and for all of my babies to come... I love you with a love that is lifetimes old. You are my inspiration, now and always.

- *AUDREY COUTO MCCLELLAND*

For Barry, the Rocket, the love of my life! Thank you for your never-wavering love, support, confidence, and inspiration. Thank you for believing in my words and my dreams. Thank you for giving me the greatest gifts of all - Audrey, Jane, Keith and Adam... and for loving them, encouraging them, and nurturing them as much as you love and encourage and nurture me. Thank you, too, for giving me five little miracles... Taylor, Madison, Andrew, Jacob, and now William... and for the miracles yet to be conceived, but whom I feel all around me.

- *SHARON K. COUTO*

Special Acknowledgments

A book of this nature, encompassing so much information – from medical to magical, from wisdom to wonder, from common-sensible to wonderfully-sensual, from technology and technique to ceremony and celebration – requires the input from many, many people. We wish to express our gratitude and thanks to the following people whom so generously gave of their time, their expertise, and their "stories":

We lovingly and deeply thank Jane Couto, our daughter/sister respectively (and Baby William's Godmother!), for listening to our idea of writing this book, and then not only sitting through hours and hours of our reading aloud excerpt upon excerpt, but for coming onboard as the very best editor who ever edited, and the very best encourager who ever encouraged. We most lovingly thank Rita Klaczynski for believing in our subject and our book from day one, and for giving us the wisdom and strength and love that only a Mom/Grandma can give; and we know that William Klaczynski, Dad/Grandpa, was all around us in spirit as we researched and wrote, sending us pink and purple balloons at every turn… and now he looks from heaven on his great-grandson and namesake, William! We also lovingly thank Florence Couto, mother-in-law/Nana, for reminding us often that babies come from "one thing, and one thing only"… and although we certainly agree, we did find some interesting and fun information that impressed even Nana! We gratefully acknowledge Michael C. Rosenberg, D.O. for his insightful comments, questions, and suggestions in reviewing our book; we extend very special thanks to Janice Kim for being the first to believe in the power of our words and in our work, and for including a preview of our book at *The Women's Showcase in New York City*; and also to Linda Maaia for her great enthusiasm in arranging a Book Club review of our manuscript, a wonderful opportunity to respond to questions and comments prior to publication! Very special and loving thanks go to Bernadette Andrews, Marianne Klaczynski, and Karen Couto for their understanding of the desires of women to bear healthy babies, and for appreciating our senses of humor in the process of explaining it; to Susan Cross and Marcie Epstein, two "new" mommies who care so profoundly about the joys and miracles of conception and motherhood that they immediately and most carefully read every detail in our manuscript and offered the most qualifiedly positive insight imaginable; and to Nicole Couto and Aimee Couto, daughters/sisters-in-law, who so generously and lovingly allowed us to delve so publicly into such personal issues as their sex lives and fertility concerns, and particularly to Aimee for believing so profoundly in the empowerment of our words that she gave us the blessed gift of Jacob during the development of this book! We especially thank Normand Poulin, Feng Shui Consultant and owner of *Living Consciously by Design*, for his meticulous review of our manuscript, and for his enthusiastic endorsement of our consistent and mindful focus of "conception affirming" spaces and energies! We most appreciate and acknowledge Susun S.Weed, author of many, many books, including *Wise Woman Herbal for the Childbearing Year*, for her passion in helping women of all ages, in all circumstances, and for taking the time to speak with us regarding preconception and fertility and allowing us to use her own very, very wise words and advice! And we offer a very special thanks to Wendy Gladding for caring deeply about our words, and for introducing us to fellow authors on their journeys to sharing our words with the world; and to Rick Couto… whom we cannot thank enough for his talents, expertise, and boundless creativity and humor in bringing our words from the manuscript to the finished work… the process certainly is like giving birth!

We also wish to sincerely thank the following people for reading our manuscript and supplying us with important feedback - some two to three times - until we got it perfect: Paula McClelland, Barbara Folgo, Jane Cotter, Sharon Waterman, Paul Lawrence, Maureen Conway, Trauti Benjamin, Liz Morgan, Nicole Navega, Sue Nasciemento, Sandra Burke, Jessica Pezzullo, Amy Pontes, Tamra Moore, Molly McClelland, Christine Davenport, Mindy McClelland, Rebecca Grady, Gretchen Fluhme, Jennifer Donnelly, Dr. Warren Ellsworth; to Lorie Muller, Jen Silva, Tammi Bannon, Cassie DiGiacomo, Marissa Saine, and Erinn Carlsten for blessing the world with Olivia, Sophia, Arianna, James, Victoria, and Chase during the development of our book; and special thanks go to Don and Karen Shortman, Bill and Renette Whitty, Susan Cary, Lorraine Maloney, Patty Whittet, and Levi Maaia for caring so deeply about our book!

And last but not least, we also express sincere gratitude to the men with whom we have conversed quite frankly and sometimes graphically in our quest for male input into deliciously smart and sexy preparation for conception: Barry Couto, Matthew McClelland, Chuck Damp, Doug Smoyer (Baby William's Godfather!), David McClelland, Johnny Johnson, Keith Couto, Adam Couto, Steven Porricelli, Dennis Klaczynski, Dimitri Gavriel, Bob Holt, Jeff Foltz, Bill Maaia; and Bob Crozier, who most succinctly explained, "*A great child is the product of a great manufacturing company* - ***the woman,*** *and the best inventory and supplies available* - ***the man****!*" **Exactly what we discuss in this book!**

There are numerous cultural, historical, preferential, religious, sexual, and sociological approaches to coupling that have always existed and will continue to exist as long as there are two human beings living on this planet. The basic need to love and to be loved takes on many forms which are accepted by those who practice them... and to these committed people who wish to bear healthy children,

Preconception Plain & Simple

celebrates the body, mind, soul, and sexuality of each potential parent and/or couple!

Contents

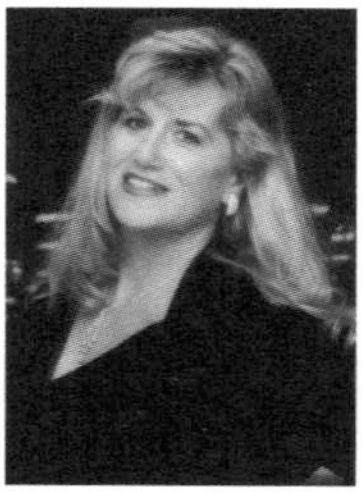

Catherine Greynolds Holden, 1959 - 2004

Our beloved cousin and friend, Cathy gave so much to her children, her family, and the world... but was called from us far too soon. She inspired us during the writing of our book with her remarkable courage, her deep concern for women and babies, her grace and beauty, and her enduring spirit. In Cathy's memory and honor, a portion of the profits from this book will be donated to Breast and Ovarian Cancer Research...

Foreword

A good beginning makes a good ending.
– *English Proverb*

You're not pregnant – yet. But you're thinking about it, which is probably why you have this book in your hands. And let's be honest… you can get pregnant without thought, care, planning, proper nutrition, or even knowing the baby's father's name - that's just the truth of it. But, and this is a *big* but… if you desire an optimal pregnancy, with the hopes and dreams of the healthiest and most intelligent child you can bear… with perfectly formed and developed heart, brain, lungs, limbs, eyesight, hearing, and speech… all of these, and more, can be influenced by the condition of your mind, body, soul, and spirit *prior* to conception! It is this *prior to conception* about which we wanted information… and as mother and daughter, we began our search!

We researched and studied every shred of information regarding preconception on which we could get our hands. Some of the information that we found on the subject of preconception comes from pregnancy resources… a chapter here… a tidbit there… or merely a page about the "dos and the don'ts" of preconception care. Some of the information comes from medical research. And still other information comes from books and conversations and chats and anecdotes and legends passed from generation to generation… culture to culture… woman to woman. So, the idea behind our book ***Preconception Plain & Simple - A Deliciously Smart and Sexy Guide in Preparing for Pregnancy!*** is to give you a comprehensive, **one-stop-resource** for every question, concern, and/or wonderment that you may have about preparing your mind, body, soul, and spirit for conception and pregnancy.

We want this time in your life to be ravishingly fun, passionately romantic, and deliciously sexy. This is a baby you're thinking about bringing into this world… what could be more extraordinary than that!?

Enjoy this book. Read it as you wish - from front to back, from back to front, a chapter here, a chapter there - *any way is suitable*. We want you to be *awed* and *ahh-ed*, and even to laugh out loud… yet we also want you to be very, very well-informed!

Enjoy, too, the icons scattered throughout this book - each indicating fun, interesting, and even magical wisdom:

Appropriately red hot, **Red Flags** highlight information for men, and… possible **rewards** for your man when he actually reads them!

Tidbits offer important and interesting "bits" of information, and also guide you to necessary preconception resources.

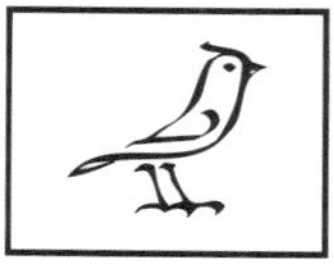

Old Wives' Tales are just what you think they are, and the ones we picked are sure to tickle your fancy!

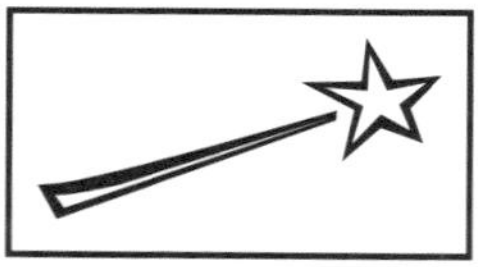

Touches of Magic will bring lots of romance, fun, and… well, *magic* to your baby-making!

Let us be your guides. The process of preparing for pregnancy is so natural, and yet also so touched with magic! Our hope is that your preconception time be blissful, beautiful, bountiful, and blessed!

Audrey Couto McClelland and Sharon K. Couto

The Conception of This Book

AUDREY'S STORY

I have always wanted children. Always dreamed of what they will look like… what I will name them (during the past 25 years I have named "my kids" dozens of times)! How many children will I have? How will I be as a mother? What will they become? The thought of having children has always been somewhere in my mind… that exciting piece of life that I couldn't wait to experience, especially after I met Matthew, who is now my husband.

Matthew and I, from day one, talked about having children. It never was a question of "if" we would; rather, it was "when" we would. But we also knew that we wanted to be a married couple for a bit, just the two of us before we brought some little ones into "our" world. Then, right after Christmas 2002, after having been married for a year and a half, it became quite apparent to us that we wanted to start preparing ourselves for a baby. Maybe it was the wonderment I saw in my brothers' eyes as they watched their daughters take their first steps… or the sight of seeing so many head-to-toe happy pregnant women out and about in New York City… or that the thought of my body getting "bigger and bigger" wasn't scary anymore, even though summer was only a few months away. Or quite possibly, the most simple truth of all, I started to get such an overwhelming feeling every time I encountered a baby - a feeling that made me say, without hesitation, "I want one."

This book came to be born on my journey to having "one". I wanted to learn how to give my body, my mind, and my soul all the nourishment, love, relaxation, and comfort that I could in preparation for having a baby. I wanted to ensure that I took all of the proper and necessary precautions in preparing my own self, preparing Matthew, and to give our future child (or children) the best chances for being a healthy human being.

But I wanted to have fun doing it... lots of it! I didn't want the baby-planning time to be filled with stress and anxiety. And as Matthew and I talked more and more about the possibility of having a baby, feelings of excitement, as well as anticipation, seemed to take over - so many things began to cross my mind: What foods should I be eating? What vitamins should I be taking? What kinds of health tests should I request from my physician? Should I chart my periods? Should we be having sex all the time? Would learning about different fertility myths and legends help? Would placing fertility symbols around our home work wonders? And I also questioned whether I should even tell people that we were thinking about "trying". All of these things (and many, many more!) entered my mind. I wanted to know what exciting, meaningful, and fun "things" Matthew and I could be doing during this preconception time!

I mean, when thinking seriously about bringing a new life into this world, shouldn't everything be covered!? And so, I immediately turned to my best friend and my best resource - my mother! She had, after all, been pregnant twice, and had experience in all of this… mind you, it was more than two decades ago… but to me, she was still my best resource – and let's be honest, what mother doesn't want to become a grandparent!?

My mother was able to share with me a few tidbits from her "time" – the 1970's – but the quarter-century that had elapsed had brought so much more information and technology that she was as comically "clueless" as I was! So my mother and I embarked upon an unexpected journey… going from bookstore to bookstore… library to library… web site to web site… looking for books and resources solely with information on everything one needs to know about preconception. Much to our own disbelief, we found very little that wasn't just medically based, and we were looking for information covering all aspects of preconception.

We did find books and web sites and resources with quick tidbits of information… a chapter here, a blurb there… but nothing to sink our teeth into. And, I'll be very honest with you, I felt odd buying books about pregnancy, even though there may have been a chapter designated for preconception in it, simply because I wasn't pregnant yet. It's like buying wedding books and magazines before you're engaged! It's an unspoken taboo! And what's the fun in reading about it if you're not fully there yet?

I wanted to find a book filled with thorough information, but extremely enjoyable to read as well… after all, this preconception time should be a fun time in one's life! I didn't want something solely medically and/or text driven.

So my mother and I spent the next few months searching through all sorts of information about preconception and pregnancy and fertility and family planning. We met with physicians, and asked dozens and dozens of women, from all different backgrounds, what they did to prepare themselves for pregnancy. The bottom line seemed to be... relax and have sex!

Hmmm... relax and have sex. Yes, the sex part I knew! But... the relax part? Relax... relax... relax. Just what would I have to do to get my body, mind, and spirit completely relaxed? Well... my mother and I began to uncover just what women have been doing for thousands of years in their preconception time. And it was fascinating! I especially wanted to find the "real" inside scoop... fun tidbits... ancient fertility secrets... fertility spells... special secret recipes... aphrodisiacs... oils... blessings... herbs... amulets... magic!

The more I learned, the more I wanted to know! And the more I knew, the more I wanted to share this information with other women.

My hope is that **Preconception Plain & Simple** *will not only aid and help women who are trying to prepare themselves for pregnancy, but also entertain them as well... bringing even more relaxation, passion, romance, and fun to this special baby-making time!*

As of today, May 6, 2003, as I write these very words, I am not pregnant yet. I am at this preconception stage with you... feeling it, living it, and wanting it to happen so very much.

Good luck to you all, and may we all have healthy, beautiful babies!

Audrey Couto McClelland

SHARON'S STORY-

On August 14, 1977, during our first wedding anniversary dinner, I sat across the dinner table from Barry, my deliciously sexy husband, and said, "Honey, I want to have a baby!"

Having previously been married and already the father of two young sons (Keith and Adam, ages 4 and 2 at the time), Barry most gently, yet most wisely answered, "Honey, babies are a lot of work... we both work full-time... a baby is a huge financial commitment... maybe we should wait for awhile..."

Of course I responded, "I know... I know..." to all of this.

But, in fact, I did not know, because I had never been near an infant in my entire life. Oh, I had baby-sat here and there during my teenage years for "big" kids, and of course I had experience with Barry's boys, but I had no siblings with infants, no friends with infants, no cousins with infants... no anybody with infants, nor had I known anyone in my circle of women who was, or had recently been, pregnant! And yes, we did both work full-time... we were both enrolled in Master's Degree programs in addition to our teaching jobs... and the time spent with Keith and Adam was very precious and very important and needed to be of the most-incredible-quality.

What I did know, though, is that I wanted to have our children raised as one family with Keith and Adam. I firmly, absolutely, resolutely knew that I did not want two separate families; and Barry, during that first anniversary heart-to-heart discussion, clearly saw the value and logic and love of this decision... and he jumped on-board (well, not that very night in the baby-making sense of the phrase... for I had some research to do)!

And so began the journey to having Audrey, our first-born daughter (and co-author of this book)!

I instinctively knew that my body should be as ready for this baby as my mind was... so the very next day I went to a bookstore on Providence's East Side in my search for books, resources, and references to help me put this baby-making plan into effect. I found little, but what I did find was a wonderful paperback book, **Nourishing Your Unborn Child***, by Phyllis S. Williams, R.N.*

Covering such topics as nutrition, healthy childbearing, and menus and recipes for pregnant women, I felt comforted that this book would help me to at least start pumping the correct and necessary nutrients into my own pre-baby body. How could it hurt?

That same day, I also found a very small "natural" food store and purchased my new book's recommended wheat germ, lecithin, whole grain flour, soybeans, and other things with which I was not at all familiar! I went home and read the ingredients and additives labels on any food and/or medication packages that had them listed. I literally devoured recipes, memorized menus, and studied the vitamin, mineral, protein, fat, etc. contents of various foods!

I also had read somewhere (and I honestly don't even remember where) about the BBT - Basal Body Temperature - method of detecting ovulation, and I purchased a Basal Body Temperature thermometer... and by the middle of October, I was pregnant! I remember taking my urine sample to our healthcare center on that crisp, fall morning, thinking, "Oh, please... please... please be positive!" And by that afternoon, my whole world was warm and wonderful and joyous with the news! Barry was working in our backyard when I announced, "Everything worked!"... then the phone calls to the new "grandparents" and aunts and uncles and friends... and finally the wonderful news about the "new baby" to Keith and Adam!

I continued to "nourish my unborn child"... devouring wonderful foods and drinks and advice... until our little bundle decided, toward the end of May, that it was time to be born – a full five weeks early! And on May 23, 1978, our precious Audrey Allison was delivered by Cesarean section... and although she was a tiny bundle (4 pounds, 9 ounces and 17 inches long), even our pediatrician was surprised at her fighting spirit!

I swore then, and still do today, that my preconception and prenatal nourishment made all the difference in my rather quick conception, and in Audrey's excellent preemie health... so when Audrey came to me in January 2003 with her own questions about preconception, I was more than happy to tell her exactly what I did to prepare for her and for my youngest daughter, Jane, now 23 years old; but I was rather surprised to find that much of what Audrey had found in "today's" information is either very clinical, very medically driven, almost frighteningly statistical, and with the word "infertility" seemingly looming everywhere… except in the advice of many obstetricians, most mothers, and virtually all grandmothers and great-grandmothers… who most wisely and most beautifully and most simply tell hopeful mothers to "just relax"!

And of course today's young women have spent their lives in whirlpools of activity, media-frenzy, instant communication, competition in sports and activities and college and graduate school admissions, demanding occupations, birth-control, and never-ever-enough time. So to tell these women to "just relax" is not like telling me to relax when I was twenty-five years old, and certainly not the same as our grandmothers being told to "just relax" and let it happen!

Yet, this is what I wanted Audrey to grasp on her journey to becoming a mother… the natural, fun, exciting, hopeful, romantic, and sexy journey… the "just relax" part of it all!

And I did have some experience in this regard, for my quick conception with Audrey had led Barry and I to believe that it would again be as expedient with our next baby… but we "tried" for six months before I became pregnant with our beautiful Jane Hillary… until I remembered and refocused on the marvel that baby-making is all about nourishment of body and spirit, lots and lots of confidence in the miraculous process, days and nights of deliciously sexy sex, and… yes… relaxation!

What I had saved all those 26+ years were two things… miraculously enough… my **Nourishing Your Unborn Child** *book and my Basal Body Thermometer… my two best friends in preparing for my beautiful babies! And although I had told Audrey this story before, this time she was listening on a higher level… a place where the past meets the future… and this simplicity was a part of the entire universe!*

It was then that the idea of our book was born… offering the most current and important medical information in preparing hopeful mothers for the healthiest babies, but also including the "ways" that women have known since time began! We found bits of information here, other bits there… we combed bookstores and libraries… we searched the web… we spoke with dozens of women and midwives and physicians… and fathers too! And we knew that what we found was important enough to be shared with other women who ***knew what to do to have a baby****, but who were unnecessarily overwhelmed by the information regarding the process!*

At first the journey was between a mother and a daughter, but what has happened over the last few months is that it has grown into a journey of womanhood.

People ask us, "What are you two doing?"

We answer, "We're writing a book!"

"About what?"

"Well… preconception. Preparing your body and spirit for a baby!"

Instantly, women step closer. They lean in. The

bond is immediate. Pretty soon we're talking about their babies, their strengths and struggles, their own journeys to having babies, sometimes traumatic... but most often miraculous! Women share their most intimate details... they ***want to share these details****. Women become disarmed. They smile or laugh or whisper or swell with tears. Women lean in to talk about their mothers and their grandmothers, their sisters and their friends, and the babies of all of these women as well!* ***When asked, women share... and it is this sharing that blends age and culture and religion and race and time.***

It is this miracle and this magic that transcends even medicine - the belief that women know so much about this baby-making power - and yet we seem to have lost such a vast piece of it in our busy, busy world.

This is what Audrey and I write about. This is what we need to share.

For what Audrey and I have discovered on this journey about babies is that all of our dreams, and the dreams of all generations - all of our pasts, our presents, and our futures - are all wrapped up in pinks and blues.

Sharon K. Couto

PART ONE

The Feet

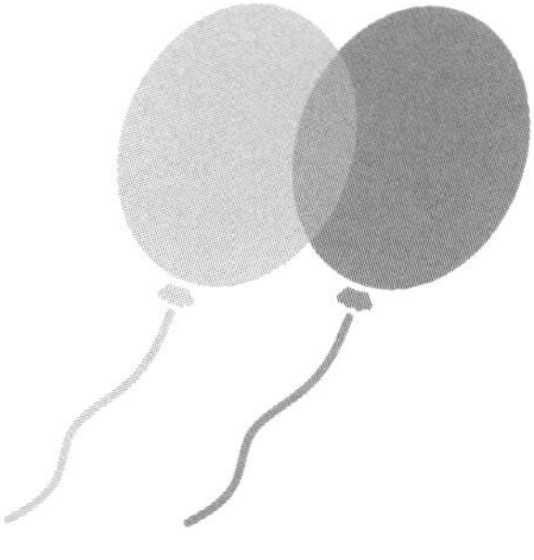

'Tis an old saying, That an ounce of prevention is worth a Pound of cure.
- BENJAMIN FRANKLIN

This is the beginning of the beginning of your journey to parenthood. What could be a more visible manifestation of your and your husband's love than a child!? This love is already vast and expansive, even though your child has not yet been conceived. This love crosses generations, continents, and cultures. This love intertwines you and your husband forever and ever and ever...

But with this love comes immense responsibility. Before this love is made visible, your *role* as a parent has already begun. It is now that you must *roll* up your sleeves... and yes, even "*roll*" down your pants (!)... to ensure that everything *with* - and *in* - your bodies is ready for take-off!

Part I of this book... what we call **The Feet** because you must be firmly grounded in health, preparation, and preventative measures prior to conception... will review every aspect of your, and your husband's, medical and ancestral histories.

The wisdom in all of this preparation and prevention is to get you to feel relaxed... to know that everything certainly is as it should be, or will be.

What you need to know is that, just like you, women and men have been both excited... and concerned... about having babies for millions and millions of years! Myths have grown around it. Medicine has grown around it. Technology has grown around it. You are not alone on this path...

Planning for a baby is the beginning of the beginning for you, but the beginning of a wondrous continuum for your baby!

CHAPTER I

Your Stories

It takes but one spark to start a fire.

- *SPANISH PROVERB*

It's so funny how life works. Many of us have spent years of our lives trying to *not* get pregnant! The hoping… the praying… the deals made with God, "Please not yet! I'll do anything!" But now the journey is a different one! You are entering into a bond, both physically and emotionally, that is the most special and miraculous bond that can be shared by two people… the conception of a baby. Just think… the magic of your relationship has become so bountiful and fulfilling that it just must multiply! Remember these words - "Children are love made visible." Well, that's true!

And so, how did all of this passion begin - from courtship… to marriage… to now, a baby carriage? As a refresher course (and a great way to enhance the mood!), relive the wild, sexy, crazy "daze" when you first met your husband*.

* The father of your future child or children may very well be your life partner, your best friend, or a sperm donor, but since the word *husband* means literally *to tend, till, cultivate, or fertilize*… for the purposes of this book, we will refer to the father as "the husband"!

Everyone has a Love Story… and it never ceases to amaze us just how excited people become when they retell it! It's as if time stops for that moment… and all other cares in the world take a back seat.

Rekindle that magic by bringing ***Your Love Story*** alive again. As funny as it may sound, *that story* is the reason you are reading this book today!

So allow yourself to slip away…
Bringing you back to that very day!

… that beautiful, enchanting day that forever changed the path of your life, and the paths of the lives of your children! Was it all part of destiny? Fate? Wild coincidence?

When was it? Where were you? Who were you with? What were you wearing? What were your first thoughts of him?

Feel like capturing it in writing!? Oh, go ahead…

Now, of course your husband will have a different spin, version, or recollection of the first time you two met. After all, he's looking through *his* own eyes! But try him out (dare ask him to put his version in writing?)! Ask *him* to bring *himself* back to that very day too... and laugh together, joke together, and compare recollections together! **How about giving him rewards for participation!?**

And now look at the two of you - thinking of having a baby! Would you ever have thought...?

For example... **Our Stories!**

SHARON

It was purely primal mating instinct (and I had 2 boy-"friends" at the time!). The first thing I saw on my future husband were his legs (in sexy, black, silky jersey shorts)! We were both teaching summer school in the summer of 1975... he was walking by, on the opposite side of a partition, which was why I could only see his legs - and I remember thinking, "If the rest of him looks as good as this..." and of course, it did, and that was it! We were married the following summer! It's been more than twenty-eight years... and yes, he still has the same great legs!

AUDREY

It was the spring of 1998 at a college house party. I can still describe the house to a "T"! I was dating someone else at the time... but as I walked into the room with one of my girlfriends, I saw the most incredibly handsome man (in a light blue button-down shirt and khaki pants) across the room. I had never seen him around campus before, so I assumed he had graduated! I remember turning to my friend and saying, "Now, why are guys like him always recent grads!?" Luckily for me, he had just been away for a year! We were married June 30, 2001... and I still think he's the most incredibly handsome man I have ever seen!

Now... (ooooh-la-la!) think back to the very first time that you and your husband *made love*... let's repeat....*made LOVE* - not *babies* (well, maybe some of you actually did "make" a baby that first time! It's been known to happen)! This is the passionate and deliciously sexy sex... the "Oh, my!... most blood-pumping, genital-swelling, earth-shaking, moon-reaching, rocketship-powered, universe-awakening lovemaking" that you must re-capture in your wonderful time of baby-preparation and baby-making! After all, making a baby is *making love*! And please, take our advice, don't write any of these particular details! The child whom you are thinking of conceiving may be reading this book some day!

And, as wildly fun and romantic as it is to bring yourself back to the very moment that you met your husband, and to the very first time that you two made love... and perhaps even to your wedding day... it's funny how we often forget to think that *we* are here - living and breathing - because two people brought *us* into this world with that same love and passion (OK... we hope!).

Yet many of us have never chronicled, or journaled, or even *discussed* the story of our own beginnings by asking questions of our own mothers and fathers (even if some of us have found the tattered baby books with the faded ink scribblings of first words, or dates of first steps)!

So while thoughts of creating a new life are dancing around in your head(s), take the time to explore your *own* beginning of life. How did *you* come to be? Obviously, none of us want to know the *gory* details of our parents' sex life (lalalalala!), but there are some wonderfully intriguing questions that you can ask both your mother and your father. You never know... you may even discover that your parents have different recollections/memories of your beginning!

So sit back and enjoy reading through... and perhaps even asking... the following questions of your mother and/or father, or anyone else who knew you as an infant. Have fun with this!

We even provided some space for you to start chronicling *your* beginning! And hey, you never know, in twenty-some-odd years(!) you may be asked the same questions by the child you are now thinking of conceiving! Enjoy…

TO YOUR MOM/DAD - MY STORY

1. Was I planned? (or as we like to say, an "Ahhhhh… " baby!)

2. Was I a surprise? (or as we like to say, an "Ohhhhh… " baby!)

3. How long had you been married or in a relationship?

4. Do you remember your conversation(s) about deciding to conceive me?

5. Did you do anything to prepare your bodies for pregnancy as we are doing now?

6. Were there any medical conditions that concerned you?

7. Had you had any miscarriages prior to conceiving me?

8. How long did it take you to conceive?

9. How "far along" were you when you found out that you were pregnant? Do you remember the date?

10. How did you find out that you were pregnant (urine test, blood test, etc...)?

11. How old were you (both Mom and Dad)?

12. What was your/*my* due date?

13. Did you feel emotionally ready for a baby? Or another baby?

14. (To your mother) How did you tell my father that you were pregnant? And how did he react?

15. How did you announce the news to my grandparents? How did they react?

16. Did you think I was a boy or a girl? Did you have Sonograms? Amniocentesis?

17. How did you come to name me?

18. What foods did you crave while you were pregnant with me?

19. Who was there on the day I was born?

20. On which day of the week was I born?

Monday's Child is fair of face,
Tuesday's Child is full of Grace,
Wednesday's Child is full of woe,
Thursday's Child has far to go…
Friday's Child is loving and giving,
Saturday's Child must work for its living,
But the Child who is born on the Sabbath Day
is wise and bonny and good and gay!

21. What was my weight? Length? Time of birth?

22. How was I received by my siblings?

23. Do you know *when* I was conceived (the actual date)?

24. *Where* was I conceived (not the "in the back seat of your father's Mustang convertible" type of information… we mean the town/city/county; state/country; continent!)?

25. In which phase was the moon on the day I was born? Very few of your parents will know this information, but it can be very interesting!… see page 193, and/or visit a web site such as **http://www.shetline.com/java/moonphase/moonphase.html** or **http://aa.usno.navy.mil/data/docs/MoonPhase.html**!

Now take the time to ask your in-laws the same questions about your husband. How did *he* come to be? Let's face it, you know he's probably not going to ask on his own! **But if he does... possible rewards!**

TO HIS MOM/DAD - HIS STORY

1. Was he planned? (or as we like to say, an "Ahhhhh..." baby!)

2. Was he a surprise? (or as we like to say, an "Ohhhhh... " baby!)

3. How long had you been married or in a relationship?

4. Do you remember your conversation(s) about deciding to conceive him?

5. Did you do anything to prepare your bodies for pregnancy as we are doing now?

6. Were there any medical conditions that concerned you?

7. Had you had any miscarriages prior to conceiving him?

8. How long did it take you to conceive?

9. How "far along" were you when you found out that you were pregnant? Do you remember the date?

10. How did you find out that you were pregnant (urine test, blood test, etc...)?

11. How old were you (both Mom and Dad)?

12. What was your/*his* due date?

13. Did you feel emotionally ready for a baby? Or another baby?

14. (To his mother) How did you tell his father that you were pregnant? And how did he react?

15. How did you announce the news to his grandparents? How did they react?

16. Did you think he was a boy or a girl? Did you have Sonograms? Amniocentesis?

17. How did you come to name him?

18. What foods did you crave while you were pregnant with him?

19. Who was there on the day he was born?

20. On which day of the week was he born?

21. What was his weight? Length? Time of birth?

22. How was he received by his siblings?

____

____

23. Do you know *when* he was conceived (the actual date)?

____

____

24. *Where* was he conceived (not the "in the back seat of his father's Mustang convertible" type of information… we mean the town/city/county; state/country; continent!)?

____

____

25. In which phase was the moon on the day he was born? Very few parents will know this information, but it can be very interesting!… see page 193, and/or visit a web site such as **http://www.shetline.com/java/moonphase/moonphase.html** or **http://aa.usno.navy.mil/data/docs/MoonPhase.html**!

____

____

SNAPSHOTS IN TIME

Take some time to look at photographs of the two of you as children… let yourself be both *awed* and *ahh-ed*… (and look on the bright side - it's a good way for you to do some extra bonding with the in-laws)!

Feel the love that leaps off of these pages! Allow your preconception time to be guided by this love - and by romance, passion, and delicious sex!

Allow your preconception time to be enhanced by your pasts… the present… and your collective future!

PHOTO OF YOU AS A CHILD

PHOTO OF YOUR HUSBAND AS A CHILD

FAMILY TREE

Ah! The mysteries and milestones and magnificence of family!

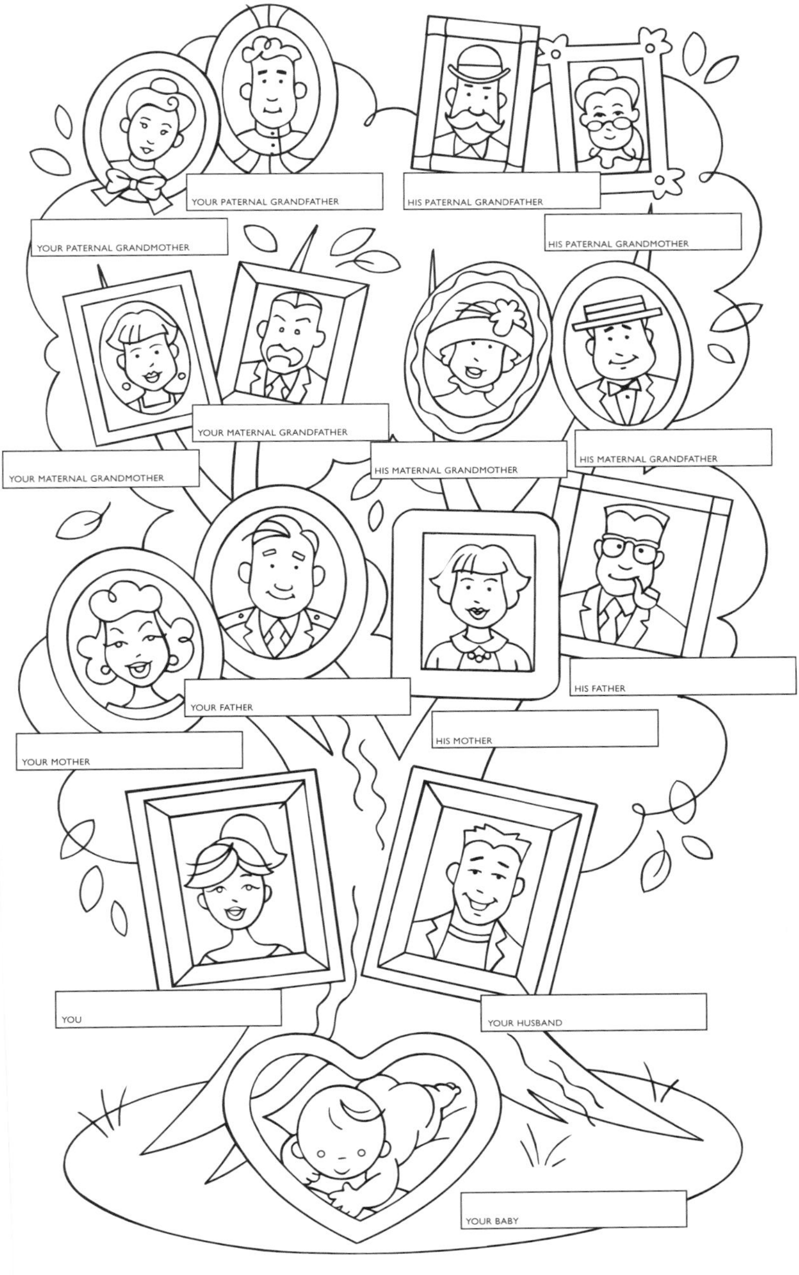

CHAPTER 2

The Medical Component- Plain & Simple

If anything is sacred, the human body is sacred.

- WALT WHITMAN

You and your husband are preparing to create a human being who will come from the most sacred places of your bodies... and the time to start taking care of your bodies is *before* you conceive.

Let's be realistic... unless your gynecologist/obstetrician/midwife is a personal friend or family member (and let's hope he/she is not your mother or father-in-law!), the chances of getting a preconception examination/appointment within the next couple of days are slim to none. And let's face it... since you and your husband have decided that you want to start preparing for a baby, you probably want to see your physician "yesterday"!

But, in the meantime, there are some important and necessary adjustments that you (and your husband - see Chapter 3: **Your Man**) can do on your own, prior to your preconception visit, that will enhance the health and well-being of both of you *and* your future baby. These are not mere suggestions... these are requirements that you cannot allow yourself to gloss over. Even if you assume or think that you are healthy - both physically and emotionally - take the following information not only for what it's worth to you, but also to your baby.

And, although baby-making is fun and exciting and sexy, this chapter is factual and medically based. We refer to this chapter as the *nuts and bolts*, or the *foundation* of this preconception time. You may even need to read this chapter, or parts of it, over and over again, as it contains far too much information to assimilate in one reading.

Remember... all *four* of your **Feet** (yours plus your husband's!) must firmly be grounded in health, preparation, and preventative mode!

So... for ease of reading, we have divided this chapter into 3 distinct parts:

1. Prior to Your Preconception Examination

2. Preconception Examination

3. Genetic Counseling (if necessary)

1. Prior to Your Preconception Examination

Deciding when to start preparing your body for pregnancy is really a personal choice. We spoke to some women who gave themselves one month... some who gave themselves six months... and still others who gave themselves one full year of preparation. Now, even though there really isn't a "correct" answer, we suggest that you give yourself at least three to four months to prepare for pregnancy. Why three to four months? Well, that gives your body enough time to adapt to any lifestyle choices that you must either start or stop. You must give yourself enough time to start thinking like a mother, for with motherhood the seesaw of responsibility tilts to your child (and fathers are not "off the hook" either... see Chapter 3). Just keep thinking to yourself what the miraculous outcome will be... a beautiful little version of both you and your husband!

And so, here we go...

1. Make sure that your Annual Physical Examination is complete, and all medical information is up-to-date!

Some short-and-sweet advice... since your General Practitioner or Family Physician is the person who most likely monitors your general health concerns, make sure that this person is aware that you are preparing to conceive a baby.

2. Start Taking Folic Acid!

It is imperative that your diet include the important nutrient *folic acid*. In fact, the United States Public Health Service recommends that all women of childbearing age should consume foods that are high in folic acid, and/or take a folic acid supplement of 400 micrograms (0.4mg) per day. If your diet already includes foods that are high in folic acid, wonderful! If not, foods that are recognized as high in folic acid are… greens such as kale, spinach, broccoli and lettuce; fruits such as oranges and melons; and wheat germ, bran, nuts and seeds.

As far as folic acid supplements, most pharmacies and/or supermarkets sell these in their vitamin sections… and the best part is that they are very tiny, and therefore not hard to swallow (which for some women is great news… no horse pills!).

> **TIDBIT** Remember that Folic Acid is a B vitamin, and is essential for cell growth and reproduction.

Now… why is folic acid so necessary to add to your body? Well, for one, folic acid has been proven to reduce spinal cord and brain birth defects (including spina bifida, a defect in which vertebrae fuse together improperly and cause the spinal cord to be exposed).

Add folic acid to your body immediately, and even recommend folic acid to all of your adult female family members and friends (even those who are not yet even thinking about having babies). The sooner you start taking folic acid, the better!

3. Stop Smoking Immediately!

Are you ready for this reality check? Women who smoke prior to pregnancy run a greater risk of infertility and miscarriage! Cigarette components such as nicotine can cause ovary damage, and also interfere with production of estrogen, and these factors alone can cause your eggs to suffer abnormalities. In addition, smoking is known to lead to low birth-weight babies, placental abnormalities, stillbirths, and higher rates of Sudden Infant Death Syndrome (SIDS)… not to mention that nicotine often causes an appetite reduction that tends to limit the intake of valuable nutrients needed to conceive, and to keep you healthy.

A WORD TO THE WISE:

Even second-hand smoke exposure can cause serious lung defects in fetuses and children... so share this information with people who love you and your future baby; and try to stay out of smoky restaurants, bars, and other areas where smoking is permitted. Also, since smoking may increase your baby's risk of Sudden Infant Death Syndrome (SIDS), use this preconception time to **stop smoking!**

If you smoke, you simply MUST "kick the habit" NOW... there are NO excuses.

And yes, we know that smoking isn't the easiest habit to quit... so really use this preconception time to get yourself into any program(s) or treatment(s) that will help you with, and through, your withdrawal - *prior* to conception.

4. Stop Drinking Alcohol!

Many women believe that alcohol consumption should cease *after* conception, but you are preparing your body *for* conception - so it's important that you start flushing your body of all alcohol, including beer, wine, and liquor. Now... we've all heard stories of the woman who drank a couple of glasses of wine each evening with dinner prior to conceiving, and even during pregnancy, and who still had the most gifted and beautiful baby of all... but what we *are* saying is that since no safe level of alcohol consumption (during pregnancy) has been established by the medical community, why not use

TIDBIT

For great alternatives to those comfy, social, and sometimes stress-relieving alcoholic beverages that you may enjoy, why not try "virgin" specialties!?

Virgin Strawberry Daiquiri
Virgin Banana Daiquiri
Virgin Bloody Mary
Virgin Piña Colada
Virgin Irish Coffee
Virgin Black Russian
Non-Alcoholic Champagne/Beer

Acquire a taste for these delectable virgin drinks during preconception... (*something* may as well be virginal!)!

your preconception time to break any addictions and/or excessive social drinking habits. If you are committed to not drinking while pregnant, why not commit this "gift" to your child three or four months (or for however long you choose) prior to pregnancy?

What we *do know* is that alcohol consumption during pregnancy is one of the greatest causes of birth defects. Drinking alcohol can cause Fetal Alcohol Syndrome (FAS) - babies with smaller heads, abnormal facial features, permanent hearing loss, learning and attention problems, skeletal malformations, and central nervous system dysfunctions (to name a few). Our thought process is... why run these risks?

5. Stop All Birth Control Methods
(*except condom use for those in the pre̲conception phase)!

Hmmm... perhaps the favorite "change" of all! We all know by now that birth control is for people who do not want to conceive. This may be the first time that you and your husband have had, or have anticipated, unprotected sex... and many women (and men!) find this exhilarating! Finally, no preparation... no worries... not a care in the world! But before you get into this deliciously sexy sex, here are some recommendations:

> **Oral Contraceptives** - *Sources vary from allowing your body anywhere from two months to one year to eliminate oral contraceptives. Simply put, progestin-only birth control pills can prevent ovulation, but they usually work by making your cervical mucus (yes... lovely thought) thick enough to prevent sperm from reaching your eggs! Combination pills, containing both estrogen and progestin, chiefly prevent your ovaries from releasing eggs altogether! How easy is this? When you're ready, just "kill" the pill!... but check with your own*

physician/midwife for his/her advice.

Spermicides *(the gels, creams, foams, vaginal suppositories, and films... most containing the not-so-sperm-friendly "nonoxynol-9"... used either alone, or with the use of a condom or diaphragm) - Recommendations range from one month to three months of discontinuing use prior to conception. Personally, we would go for the two or more months of discontinuing use, as you don't want any "sperm killers" lurking around your cervix!*

> **TIDBIT** It is estimated that over the course of one year, about 29 out of 100 typical couples who rely on spermicides alone will have an accidental pregnancy!

Intrauterine Device (IUD) *- Definitely (and obviously) have your IUD removed before attempting to conceive. Since an IUD is 97% effective in preventing pregnancy... we're "pretty" sure you'll want it removed if you are seriously considering conceiving!*

A WORD TO THE WISE:

Since most couples must rely on a contraceptive during preconception time, recommendations include: 1) using a condom* (alone... without spermicides... because you certainly don't want nonoxynol-9 "knocking" on your cervix door!); or 2) using a diaphragm (again, no spermicides!) while waiting for your preconception exam.

---

6. Stop Douching!

Yes, we want to feel clean, and smell really, really nice "down there"... but the National Women's Health Information Center offers some

> **TIDBIT** A sperm-friendly vaginal environment means avoiding all douches, scented tampons, vaginal deodorant sprays, and even... yes... saliva!

advice on douching - DON'T! Research shows that douching decreases your conception chances because the process "washes" out your wonderfully fertile cervical fluids… yes, the same fluids that help your husband's sperm reach their goal! Other research even suggests a link between frequent douching and low-birth weight babies. Hmmm…

7. Stop Using Illegal Substances Immediately

(cocaine, marijuana, ecstasy, amphetamines, heroin, LSD, etc.) Ughhh…! And yes, we'll do that again… Ughhh!

If you are currently using any of the above substances, either casually or otherwise, please… please… please… don't even start thinking of having a baby until you are "clean". Honestly. You must seek the advice of your healthcare provider, physician, and/or a drug counselor. We're not even going to feed into your denial, or enable you in any way, by suggesting that you just stop using these substances while trying to conceive. Drug use is the ultimate act of selfishness and irresponsibility to your baby… and really to society as a whole. If you have read what smoking and drinking alcohol can possibly do to your baby… just imagine the complete and utter damage and destruction caused by drugs. Period.

TIDBIT As reported on sciencedaily.com… a study released by Yale University cites that cocaine use during pregnancy causes attention/memory defects, impulsivity, and learning deficits in children. Many drug-using mothers (heroin, cocaine, marijuana, PCP) give birth to drug-addicted babies, who then suffer conditions such as tremors, poor coordination, and feeding problems.

8. Limit Caffeinated Products

(coffee, tea, chocolate, and soft drinks)

Although no research is definitive in the caffeine category, some studies indicate that 3 or more cups of coffee per day (300 mg. caffeine - the equivalent of 8 cans of soda or 6 cups of tea) may decrease a woman's chances of conception by as much as 27%. Wow!

AUDREY'S QUANDARY!

For me, even as I write this book, this is a tough one! I thought I could not live without my morning large (equivalent to probably 4 regular cups!) black coffee... could not live, never mind try to function throughout my day! The first day that I tried to go without it, I had a severe headache by lunch... but, even though days of beating headaches followed, I was able to wean myself off the caffeine. OK, maybe I have cheated a tiny bit - but I have switched to a morning decaffeinated large, black coffee... and I have replaced my lunchtime diet coke with water (even better for my skin!).

What really got me the most motivated to change my ways was reading that three or more cups of coffee per day may affect fertility. Ouch! That frightened me... and again, like smoking and alcohol consumption, it's just better to start weaning away from these products prior to pregnancy, during pre-conception time.

The focus of a healthy baby tends to take your mind off of YOU - which also leads to an unselfish, more relaxed approach to baby-making!

9. Assess Your Calcium, Iron, and Zinc Intake!

That's right… take a good look at your nutrient and vitamin intake, and assess if you are getting enough calcium, iron, and zinc. These are three crucial nutrients to consider in preparing for pregnancy. In fact, begin the practice of reading labels during preconception!

CALCIUM - *Preparation for pregnancy includes making sure that your bones are healthy enough to sustain a pregnancy. We all know those commercials - "Milk… It Does a Body Good." Well, the National Institute of Health suggests that non-pregnant women require 1000mg of calcium per day (three to four servings from the milk, yogurt, and cheese [all types] group), but don't discount such foods as (yummy!) canned sardines, canned salmon, and collard greens!*

> **TIDBIT** Since an estimated 90% of American women do not get the recommended daily allowance of calcium in their daily diets, keep in mind that foods such as corn tortillas, ice cream and frozen yogurt, fortified waffles, and tofu contain calcium! Yum!

IRON - *We all know that we usually feel extra tired and run down during our periods… well, that's because our periods rob our bodies of its iron. We need the trace mineral iron in order to produce much needed hemoglobin, the powerful oxygen-carrier in our red blood cells! Since you cannot afford to be exhausted during your baby-making time (all that delicious sex!), increase your iron intake by eating lean meats, poultry, shellfish, and iron-enriched breads, pastas, and cereals.*

ZINC - *You may be surprised to learn that zinc has been known to increase vaginal lubrication, as* *well as to decrease PMS symptoms - but it does! Who would have thought? And that's not all... a healthy zinc intake also leads to larger and healthier babies (something all of us want, just as long as the baby isn't, oh, a 15-pounder)! Increase your intake of lean beef, pork, lamb, dark chicken meat (animal proteins), peanut butter, oysters, crab, cashews, almonds, and legumes in order to ensure proper zinc levels!*

10. Exercise, Weight, and Stress!

OK... what woman likes to *think* about, never mind *talk* about exercise, weight, and stress!? We'll try to be realistic here - if you're overweight, or just trying to lose those last 5 pounds - you already know it. If you exercise too much, too little, or not at all - you already know it. If stress impacts your life in any way (and if it doesn't, we'd like to meet you and learn your secrets!), only you can determine its impact on your planned pregnancy.

Every pregnancy source available will tell you either to lose weight or gain weight, exercise more or less, and even provide weight charts and graphs as supplemental resources... but these are such personal issues for women, and you alone know what you must do in the weight and exercise category to increase your chances for an optimal, healthy pregnancy. Dig deeply from within and be honest with yourself. Amazing changes are often made once we look at ourselves as *mothers*. And as far as stress, in **Part II - The Wings,** we will do our best to get you to eat and dance and bathe and scent yourself into relaxation!

Again, use this preconception time to reflect on your *excuses* for not exercising, not eating properly, or not relaxing... and then get yourself pro-active in making the healthiest version of you - if not for yourself, then for your baby! And also, don't hesitate to ask for help if you need it. Sometimes we do need motivators who are going to pick us up when we're down and rally us to victory. Rely on the support of those who love you!

Set your goals... be realistic... and go for it! Hey, perhaps your new focus on healthy exercise and weight changes (as a Mommy!) will help you relax enough to relieve some of those life-related stresses, as well as to get your body all the more ready for delicious sex and conception!

11. Visit Your Dentist!

A WORD TO THE WISE:
Whitening treatments, bonding, and X-rays should be avoided during pregnancy... so try to take care of these needs during your preconception time!

Your teeth are a part of who you are! Pregnancy may exacerbate common dental problems (yes, the not-so-lovely nuisances of increased salivation, bleeding gums, and extra plaque, all brought on by extra blood flow and increased estrogen levels!)... so it is best to take care of those "pearly whites" prior to conception!

Schedule an appointment with your dentist for a thorough cleaning during your preconception time... and promise (each day!) to brush twice with a fluoride toothpaste and floss away food particles that cause harmful bacteria and plaque. While you're at it, practice putting only excellent foods into your mouth (not the sugary stuff that leads to tooth decay)!

OLD WIVES' TALE: For each baby, a mother loses another tooth!

12. Be Aware of Environmental Issues!

Be aware that exposure to radiation can not only cause fertility problems in both men and women, but can cause birth defects as well... and cleaning substances, lawn chemicals, and some paints and pesticides are possible home hazards that may affect fertility and pregnancy. Further, consider that some of your hobbies may expose you to harmful substances - these include exposure to paint thinners, lacquers, varnish removers, plastics, and lead.

It is common sense to know that you should always avoid exposure to hazardous chemicals, toxic substances (such as lead and pesticides), and solvents both at work and at home... but like exercise, weight, and stress, only *you* can make the very tough decisions whether or not you can alter the way you have always lived. We cannot tell you to quit your job, or to relocate... just like we cannot tell you that you must hire a personal trainer... but these are things that you should discuss not only with your husband, but with your physician as well. Perhaps there are smaller changes that can be implemented in your life to avoid environmental "concerns"... such as the ventilation of dangerous areas, use of rubber gloves or surgical masks, or avoidance of activities/hobbies during active preconception and/or pregnancy.

> **TIDBIT** The magazine CHILD (Dec./Jan. 2004) cites a great web site to look to for such concerns... so if you have any questions regarding environmental risks, go to http://www.motherisk.org. Check it out!

All leading to the much anticipated...

2. Preconception Examination

OK... this is probably going to be the moment when the entire baby-making idea seems to actually be REAL! You're meeting with your gynecologist... your midwife... your healthcare provider... and now the serious questions and tests should be addressed. You may be excited... nervous... scared... anxious...

euphoric, but try to relax. This visit will put to rest, or address, any situations that could complicate a pregnancy… and give you the "green light" to fertility!

This is your time to sit and to have your physician/midwife's undivided attention. This may even be the first time you have had a serious discussion about having a baby with someone other than your husband! Enjoy! And please try to *not* be a hypochondriac at this time… that certainly is not our intention with the following medical discussion! We have tried to make this visit "Plain and Simple" for you so that you will be very prepared… for, in the words of Ralph Waldo Emerson… "*The right performance of this hour's duties will be the hours or best preparation for the ages that follow.*" And as far as your husband… well, in the words of Nolan Richardson, "*Preparation prevents piss-poor performance!*"

And please remember… your physician/midwife will be getting almost as intimate with you as your husband will! So, if you do not feel completely at ease, comfortable, relaxed, and confident with this person, get a new physician/midwife immediately! We have heard horror stories from women who were made to feel downright "stupid" if they asked questions… or who were "dismissed" if they dared to bring up something "new" that they had read… or who met with physicians on-call more often than they met with their own physician! Still others have become virtual "best buds" with their physicians/midwives. A "happy medium" situation is something that you might have to spend some time seeking, and the preconception time is the perfect time in which to do it!

And so… what follows is a list of questions that address personal information, existing conditions, and/or genetic diseases/conditions that (if necessary) may, can, and will be treated prior to, and/or during your pregnancy. We have developed the following questionnaire for you to use as a guide while discussing pregnancy with your physician/midwife.

Don't be frightened or intimidated by the thoroughness of the next few pages. Read through the following questions/comments... and actually bring the questionnaire to your preconception visit so that you can discuss any question(s)/comment(s) that apply specifically to you, or that concern you.

Remember that the information we are providing will be most beneficial to you if you prepare yourself *prior* to your visit... then you will know *exactly what you need to discuss* with your physician/midwife. Use the time *prior* to your preconception examination to "dig around" for your medical histories so that you are completely prepared for your appointment. You don't want to sit with your physician/midwife saying, "I don't know... I don't remember"... to very important questions and information that may affect your pregnancy.

Engage in and enjoy an open and honest conversation with your physician/midwife! This is a *baby* you're getting ready to start trying for! Smile! Be happy! And just relax!

OK... here we go!

GENERAL QUESTIONS/COMMENTS

Tear-off checklist is available for your convenience - see Appendix, page 205!

My birth date is ______________________ (I am ___ years old).

My husband's birth date is _______________ (he is ___ years old).

This is our first time trying to conceive a baby ☐ yes ☐ no.

We plan to actively start trying _________________ (month/year).

We have been trying to conceive for ___ months/years.

The date of my last menstrual period was ____________________.

My periods are regular / irregular and come approximately every ________ days.

We are currently using ______________ as a birth control method.

I (we) have used (birth control methods) ____________, _________________, _________________ in the past.

Date(s): ____

I have been pregnant ____ times.

Date(s): ____

Weight of baby(ies): ___________________________________

Delivery Method(s): ___________________________________

Complications: ____

Premature births: ______________________________________

I have had ____ miscarriage(s).

Date(s): ____

I have had ____ ectopic pregnancy(ies).
Date(s): ______________________________

I have had ____ abortion(s) - *(be sure to tell your physician where, when, and by whom, so that your physician will be able to determine if a pregnancy may be affected in any way)*.

My last Pap Smear was ______________________ (date).

My last Mammogram was ______________________ (date).

Can you recommend an excellent preconception/pre-natal woman's vitamin supplement? And a supplement for my husband?

____

____

Do we need to change our diets in any way? (*in other words, we currently follow Atkins, Zone, Vegan, Lactose Intolerant, Blood Type, etc.*)

Do we need to stop taking any prescribed medications? (*bring a list of all prescribed medications with you, including*):

Anti-Acids
Anti-Anxiety
Antibiotics
Anti-Coagulants
Anti-Depressants
Anti-Gas
Anti-Inflammatory
Anti-Itch Products

> **TIDBIT** Some medications used to treat diseases such as arthritis, fungal infections, ulcerative colitis, and seizures can affect the quantity and quality of sperm... so discuss this with your physician if it applies to you! Remember that, in most cases, the effects of these medications are reversible when stopped!

- Appetite Suppressants
- Birth Control
- Blood Pressure Medications
- Cancer Medications
- Cholesterol Medications
- Cold Medications
- Diuretics
- Fungal and/or Yeast Infections
- Hemorrhoid Treatments
- Indigestion Medications
- Laxatives
- Nasal Sprays
- Pain Medications
- Sedatives
- Seizure Medications
- Steroids

Yes, bring a list of *everything*!

Can we continue taking over-the-counter medications? *(bring a list of all over-the-counter medications that you use - refer to above list)*

Can we continue taking herbal products? *(bring a list of all herbal products that you currently use; for examples, St. John's Wort may adversely affect sperm, and herbs such as Pennyroyal and Tansy actually stimulate uterine contractions, which you may not want!)*

I was adopted ☐ yes ☐ no.

My husband was adopted ☐ yes ☐ no.

Will my work environment (explain)… our home environment (explain)… or my hobbies (explain) harm my chances of conceiving and/or having a healthy baby? *(bring a list of all substances with which you come into contact, or inhale)*

Will my husband's work environment (explain)… or his hobbies (explain) harm my chances of conceiving and/or having a healthy baby? *(bring a list of all substances with which your husband comes into contact, or inhales)*

My blood type is ________.

My husband's blood type is ________.

I have had a Blood Transfusion ☐ yes ☐ no.

Date(s) ______________________________

Explain ______________________________

Should I be concerned about toxoplasmosis? (*parasitic infection spread through cat feces and/or rare meat that can increase risks of fetal mental retardation, blindness, and can lead to possible miscarriage*)

I have a history of problems with anesthesia ☐ yes ☐ no.

Explain ______________________________

VACCINATIONS YOU MAY NEED

If possible, bring your vaccination record or history. Your record should indicate that you have been immunized against the following (*most of these you received during infancy or childhood, or before you started school!*):

Chicken Pox
Hepatitis A
Hepatitis B
HIB (Haemophilus Influenza Type B)
Measles
Mumps
PCV (Pneumococcal Conjugate Vaccine)
Polio
Rubella

Should I receive a "flu shot" against influenza?

Should I receive a Chicken Pox vaccination? (*if you've never had Chicken Pox, 1 to 2% of babies whose mothers contract Chicken Pox while pregnant - especially between 8 to 20 weeks - are born with 1 or more birth defects... including eye problems, poor growth, delayed development*)

> **TIDBIT** Most sources suggest waiting at least one month after being immunized for Chicken Pox before trying to conceive.

Should I receive a vaccination to prevent Hepatitis B? (*condition that results in liver disease that can be passed to baby*)

Should I receive a Lyme Disease vaccination, if available? (*a serious bacterial infection caused by a tick bite infection... can be passed to baby; although rare, it can make a woman more likely to miscarry*)

Should I receive a Tetanus Booster? (*tetanus is caused by bacterial toxins that infect open wounds, which, in turn, can lead to Lock Jaw and muscle spasms*)

TESTING THAT COULD BE DONE

> **TIDBIT** Cytomegalovirus (CMV)- part of the herpes virus group; includes the viruses that cause Chicken Pox, mononucleosis ("Mono"), and herpes, and is spread through urine, blood, saliva, tears, semen, breast milk, and vaginal fluids.

Should I be tested for Cystic Fibrosis? (*a genetic disease that causes thick cervical mucus, blocking entry of sperm into cervix*)

Should my husband be tested for Cystic Fibrosis? (*can cause sterility in men*)

Should I be tested for Cytomegalovirus? (*can cause miscarriage and developmental problems in baby*)

Should I be tested for Fifth Disease? (*caused by Parvovirus B-19, a pregnant woman can spread the virus to her fetus, resulting in possible miscarriage in early pregnancy*)

Should I be tested for Fragile "X" Syndrome? (*defective X-Chromosome, causing mild retardation*)

Should I be tested for Group B Strep? (*strep can affect baby in the birth canal during delivery*)

Should I be tested for Tuberculosis? (*bacterial infection that can spread through the lymph nodes and bloodstream to any organ in your body*)

My ethnic background is ______________________________.

My husband's ethnic background is ______________________.

If you are of Eastern European Jewish decent: Should I receive a Tay-Sachs Disease blood test? (*heritable metabolic disorder causing dementia, paralysis, blindness*)

If you are of African American decent: Should I receive a Sickle Cell Disease blood test? (*inherited blood disorder causing bone marrow to produce red blood cells with defective hemoglobin, reducing blood flow to the body*)

> **TIDBIT** Hemoglobin is the protein in red blood cells that carries oxygen and nutrients to all parts of the body.

If you are of African American or Southern Asian decent: Should I receive a Thalassemia blood test? (*inherited blood disorder that affects the ability to produce hemoglobin*)

If you are 35 years old or older... or if there is a family history: Should I receive genetic screening and counseling to discuss chromosomal defects such as Down Syndrome? *(genetic condition causing delays in physical and intellectual development)*

YOUR PERSONAL MEDICAL HISTORIES

You must make your physician/midwife aware of any medical conditions that you or your husband have, or have had, and you must be totally honest. You cannot be embarrassed by any of these conditions and/or questions. Again, the well-being of your future baby depends upon your honesty during your **Preconception Visit**. Allow your physician to alleviate any fears... and by being an intelligent and caring person, don't let any stone go unturned.

Take a look at the following list of conditions that either of you have, may have, or have had, as these may need to be managed properly during your pregnancy. Check any that apply to you and/or your husband:

☐ you **ABORTIONS** - if performed improperly, could cause infertility

☐ you **ANOVULATION** - a fertility cycle without ovulation, sometimes caused by stress, excessive exercise, travel, illness, drug use

☐ you **DIETHYLSTILBESTROL** (drug known as DES) - taken by women from 1930 - 1971, has caused reproductive problems in daughters of women who took this drug

☐ you **ENDOMETRIOSIS** - inflammation of the inside lining of the uterus

☐ you **OVARIAN CYST** - small fluid-filled sac that grows in the ovaries

☐ you **PELVIC INFLAMMATORY DISEASE (PID)** - caused by bacteria that can affect the uterus, fallopian tubes, and ovaries; resulting from ruptured appendix, non-sterile abortion, but mostly from Sexually Transmitted Diseases (STDs)

☐ you **POLYCYSTIC OVARIAN SYNDROME (PCO)** - characterized by multiple ovarian cysts and increased androgen; can cause infertility

~

☐ you ☐ him **ACNE** - side-effects of medications (ex: Acutane - recommended to stop using one month prior to conception… can cause miscarriage and birth defects)

☐ you ☐ him **ALLERGIES** - possible side effects of medications

☐ you ☐ him **ANEMIA** - can reduce amount of oxygen to baby

☐ you ☐ him **ASTHMA** - possible side effects of medications

☐ you ☐ him **CANCER** - side effects of medications/radiation

☐ you ☐ him **CYSTIC FIBROSIS** - genetic disorder that could lead to lung disease, infertility, and/or sterility

☐ you ☐ him **DIABETES** - can cause birth defects, and increase risk of miscarriage and stillbirth

☐ you ☐ him **DIGESTIVE PROBLEMS** (examples: Crohn's Disease/Colitis/Ileitis, ulcers) - possible side effects of medications

☐ you ☐ him **EATING DISORDERS** (Anorexia, Bulimia) - nutritional deficiencies can harm unborn child

☐ you ☐ him **EPILEPSY** - possible side effects of medications

☐ you ☐ him **FRAGILE "X" SYNDROME** - carried by the mother, can cause mental retardation

☐ you ☐ him **GENITAL WARTS** - caused by Human Papilloma Virus (HPV), can lead to cervical cancer or cancer of the penis

☐ you ☐ him **GONORRHEA/CHLAMYDIA** - can increase risk of infertility, ectopic (tubal) pregnancies, and sterility in men

☐ you ☐ him **HEPATITIS A, B, C** - can be harmful to mother and baby

☐ you ☐ him **HERPES** - can be harmful or fatal to baby

☐ you ☐ him **HIGH BLOOD PRESSURE** - can cause placental problems and fetal growth retardation

☐ you ☐ him **HIV/AIDS** - run the risk of infecting baby

☐ you ☐ him **HYPERTENSION** - can affect amounts of blood/nutrients that baby receives

☐ you ☐ him **KIDNEY DISEASE** - can increase risk of fetal poor growth, or death

☐ you ☐ him **LIVER DISEASE** - can be caused by Hepatitis C

☐ you ☐ him **LUPUS** - can increase risk of miscarriage and pre-term labor; sometimes flares up during pregnancy

☐ you ☐ him **MENTAL ILLNESS** - possible side effects of medications

☐ you ☐ him **MIGRAINES** - side effects of medications (ex: Imitrex - recommended to stop two to three months prior to conception)

☐ you ☐ him **OVULATION/HORMONAL DISORDERS** - can be caused by excessive exercise, eating disorders, smoking, or stress

☐ you ☐ him **PHENYLKETONURIA (PKU)** - managed properly, special diet prevents mental retardation and birth defects

☐ you ☐ him **RHEUMATOID ARTHRITIS** - symptoms sometimes *remiss* during pregnancy!

☐ you ☐ him **SEIZURES** - some medications can increase risk of birth defects

☐ you ☐ him **SURGERIES/CHEMOTHERAPY/RADIATION** - especially uterine… can cause miscarriage or premature birth, and can affect fetal development; as for your husband, any surgeries to the urogenital area should be brought to the attention of your physician, as scar tissue can cause problems with sterility

☐ you ☐ him **SYPHILIS** - can affect baby in the uterus or during delivery, causing birth defects; can lead to sterility in men

☐ you ☐ him **THYROID DISEASE** - although thyroid medications appear to be safe during pregnancy, check to make sure doses are proper

☐ you ☐ him **URINARY TRACT INFECTIONS** - can cause premature birth

☐ you ☐ him **YEAST INFECTIONS** - can become exacerbated during pregnancy

Other(s)

____

____

____

____

YOUR FAMILY MEDICAL HISTORIES

Again, take this preconception time to "dig" for information! Do whatever you must do to research your family histories! Call Mom... Dad... brother... sister... Grandma... Grandpa... aunt... uncle - anyone who can provide you with the information you are seeking! If you're not ready to tell why you're asking (not that they won't be able to figure it out!)... tell them you need the information for an insurance policy! See how long that excuse works!

Be aware if there is a **Family History** (maternal and paternal) of the following - in either **YOUR FAMILY** or **HIS FAMILY**:

☐ your family ☐ his family **ADDICTIONS**

Explain: ______________________________

☐ your ☐ his **ANEMIA**

Explain: ______________________________

☐ your ☐ his **ASTHMA, TUBERCULOSIS,** or any lung disease

Explain: ______________________________

☐ your ☐ his **CANCER** (examples: cervical, breast, prostate, testicular)

Explain: ______________________________

☐ your ☐ his **CARDIAC/NEURAL TUBE DEFECTS**

Explain: ______________________________

☐ your family ☐ his family **CEREBRAL PALSY**

Explain: ______________________________

☐ your ☐ his **CLEFT LIP/PALATE**

Explain: ______________________________

☐ your ☐ his **CONGENITAL ADRENAL HYPERPLASIA**

Explain: ______________________________

☐ your ☐ his **CROHN'S DISEASE**

Explain: ______________________________

☐ your ☐ his **CYSTIC FIBROSIS**

Explain: ______________________________

☐ your ☐ his **DIABETES**

Explain: ______________________________

☐ your ☐ his **DIETHYLSTILBESTROL (DES)**
(my mother took in 19__)

Explain: ______________________________

☐ your ☐ his **DIGESTIVE PROBLEMS**

Explain: ______________________________

☐ your ☐ his **DOWN SYNDROME/MENTAL RETARDATION**

Explain: ______________________________

☐ your ☐ his **EPILEPSY**

Explain: ______________________________

☐ your ☐ his **HEART DISEASE**

Explain: ______________________________

☐ your ☐ his **HEMOPHILIA A/BLEEDING DISORDERS**

Explain: ______________________________

☐ your ☐ his **HEPATITIS/LIVER DISEASES**

Explain: ______________________________

☐ your ☐ his **HIGH BLOOD PRESSURE**

Explain: ______________________________

☐ your ☐ his **HUNTINGTON'S DISEASE**

Explain: ______________________________

☐ your ☐ his **KIDNEY DISEASE**

Explain: ______________________________

☐ your family ☐ his family **LUPUS**

Explain: ____

☐ your ☐ his **MENTAL ILLNESS**

Explain: ____

☐ your ☐ his **MENTAL RETARDATION**

Explain: ____

☐ your ☐ his **MIGRAINES**

Explain: ____

☐ your ☐ his **MISCARRIAGE**

Explain: ____

☐ your ☐ his **MULTIPLE BIRTHS**

Explain: ____

☐ your ☐ his **MUSCULAR DYSTROPHY**

Explain: ____

☐ your ☐ his **PHENYLKETONURIA (PKU)**

Explain: ____

☐ your ☐ his **POLYCYSTIC KIDNEY DISEASE**

Explain: ______________________________

☐ your ☐ his **PREMATURE OVARIAN FAILURE** (cessation of menstruation before the age of 40)

Explain: ______________________________

☐ your ☐ his **SICKLE CELL ANEMIA**

Explain: ______________________________

☐ your ☐ his **SPINA BIFIDA/SPINE DEFECTS**

Explain: ______________________________

☐ your ☐ his **TAY-SACHS DISEASE**

Explain: ______________________________

☐ your ☐ his **THALASSEMIA**

Explain: ______________________________

☐ your ☐ his **THYROID DISEASE**

Explain: ______________________________

☐ your ☐ his **VASO VAGAL REACTION**

Explain: ______________________________

Other(s) explain:

☐ your family ☐ his family ____________________

☐ your ☐ his ____________________

☐ your ☐ his ____________________

☐ your ☐ his ____________________

☐ your ☐ his ____________________

☐ your ☐ his ____________________

☐ your ☐ his ____________________

☐ your ☐ his ____________________

☐ your ☐ his ____________________

3. Genetic Counseling

If it has been determined by your physician that you may benefit from genetic counseling, don't hesitate to contact a genetic counselor (whom often is referred by your physician). He/she will work with you and/or your family(ies) to help you gain the knowledge to record your family histories, help interpret test results, alleviate fears, and provide information to find resources with which to deal with the specific conditions.

An excellent resource in genetic counseling information is the March of Dimes - www.modimes.org. Your local chapter will have a wealth of information on genetic service centers in your area. Rely on this wonderful organization!

Whether or not you need further tests, information, or counseling… remember the words of Rene Dubois - "Each human being is unique, unprecedented, unrepeatable."

Your bodies and your babies deserve the best possible chances, which is precisely why you are reading this book!

Bravo!

CHAPTER 3

Your Man!

Every man is the builder of a temple, called his body.

- *Henry David Thoreau*

Well, we can't do it without them, that's for sure! It's the union of the two of you that will create your baby. And again, if you want an optimal pregnancy, with the best chances of having a healthy baby, your husband should assess what *he* brings to this reproduction fun (other than the obvious!).

What many men don't understand is that they are just as important to this preconception time as you are. According to ***Men's Reproductive Health*** (October 1999), "The reproductive health of women can hinge on the support and participation of their partners, yet the involvement of men in the reproductive health decision

> **TIDBIT** (or perhaps Tid**BIG**!): "An erection begins with psychological arousal and/or physical stimulation. A substance called nitric oxide is then released into the muscle cells of the penis, causing the muscle tissue to relax and expand, like a sponge into water. As the muscle tissue relaxes, in-flow of blood into the penis increases, producing an increase in both girth and length of the penis. This results in the trapping of blood that normally flows out of the penis and back into circulation." Dr. J. Francois Eid (see page 64)
>
> Hmmm... all of this needs to occur to bring us to ecstasy and/or conceive a child!? Yes!

process has only recently been given serious attention." But let's get real! Honestly, what man willingly reads books on pregnancy… never mind jumps up from dinner and says, "Gee, Honey… I hope my sauna usage at the gym last night didn't increase my scrotum temperature too dramatically! Do you think that could affect our chances of conceiving?"

We mean, it's almost laughable! And yet, as "lovely" as it sounds for his scrotum temperature to rise, it is a common cause for *low sperm count* in men. And so, just as it is important for you to think like a Mother, your husband must learn to think like a Father, putting the needs of his future children… let's just say it… FIRST!

So, ladies… take the "bull by the horns" - literally - and ask your husband to read this chapter. If you must, offer him some **rewards for reading…** you two determine the appropriate rewards, of course!

1. Physician Visit!

Schedule an appointment for your husband's Annual Physical Examination. **Extra rewards for him if he schedules his own appointment!** During his examination, your husband should make sure that he tells his physician that you and he are going to be trying to conceive a baby soon. His physician may have a wealth of information to pass along! **Even more rewards if your husband brings this information home!**

2. Ask, Beg and Drag (and we're not on the Sex chapter yet)!

Set up a date night (how sexy is this!?… going over your medical histories together) to review all of the information in preparation for your **Preconception** Examination in **Chapter 2, The Medical Component!**

And then ask him, beg him, or drag him to the actual

appointment with the physician/midwife who will be guiding both of you during your preconception time and eventual pregnancy (this is particularly important for men with genetic risk factors). In the case that your physician is a dead ringer for Brad Pitt (ohh… we wish!), your ex-boyfriend, or looks and sounds just like your mother, your husband may request that you find another physician/midwife! Seriously though, if your husband doesn't feel comfortable with the person (or persons) with whom you have made appointments, give him the love, support, and courtesy to find another provider together. Remember that this person will be poking… pulling… prodding… deciding… delving… and dealing with you, your husband, and your baby for a minimum of nine months! Period.

3. Preferably NO Smoking (Be Good To Your Sperm)!

We should say absolutely NO SMOKING, but we're going to say PREFERABLY NO SMOKING because you know and we know that he is the only one who can dig deeply enough to make this lifestyle change. But if he has trouble snuffing the "butts", let him know **(rewards if he is reading this!)** that studies suggest that a father who smokes even *before* conception is dramatically increasing his future baby's chances of developing leukemia… not to mention that smoking can damage the motility of sperm - something that men certainly do not want to mess with!

4. "Watch" the Alcohol Consumption!

OK ladies, this is a tricky topic. We don't want you to be frightened, nervous, or even the big "B" - bitchy - about your husband having a

TIDBIT

According to the U.S. Department of Agriculture and the U.S. Department of Health and Human Services, "moderate" drinking is defined as 2 drinks per day for most men… and a "standard" drink size is considered 12 oz. of beer, 5 oz. of wine, or 1.5 oz. of 80 proof distilled spirits.

couple of beers... but it is important to note that consistent alcohol consumption (and most sources list "consistent" alcohol consumption as two to three drinks per day) can cause low birth weight babies. Now again, we don't want to go into lecture-mode, but you know if your husband has a serious drinking problem… and it doesn't come down to how many drinks he consumes while watching Monday Night Football! But for the purposes of a healthy baby, heavy alcohol consumption in men is known to depress both sperm count and testosterone levels… causing, in the most serious consequences, hormonal deficiencies, sexual dysfunction, and infertility. What guy wants this?

5. Stop Using Illegal Substances (cocaine, heroin, ecstasy, marijuana, LSD, etc.)

You know that the *individual* him-or-herself is the only one who can make lifestyle choices such as smoking, drinking, overeating, exercising too much or too little… but abusing illegal substances goes beyond the aforementioned decisions. If your husband chooses to abuse his body and mind, spend money on illegal substances, as well as break the law, perhaps you should assess whether he is father material…? This is not intended to be insulting or judgmental - but illegal substances are the main causes of crime, drained finances, and spousal/child abuse. Just take this to heart with openness and non-denial. The fact that these substances are known to lower sperm count and increase infertility are the *least* of your problems. Enough said.

6. Over-the-Counter Substances, Medications, and Prescriptions!

It is important to discuss the use of your husband's medications with your physician before you conceive. You don't want anything in his system that could affect the health of your baby… and to be on the safe side, don't leave anything out. Ask his healthcare provider (or have *him* ask) about the following:

Anti-Acids
Anti-Anxiety Medications
Antibiotics
Anti-Coagulants
Anti-Depressants
Anti-Gas Medications
Anti-Inflammatory Medications
Anti-Itch Products
Appetite Suppressants
Blood Pressure Medications
Cancer Medications
Cholesterol Medications
Cold Medications
Diuretics
Fungal and/or Yeast Infections
Hemorrhoid Treatments
Indigestion Medications
Laxatives
Nasal Sprays
Pain Medications
Seizure Medications
Sedatives
Steroids
Other(s)

7. Start Taking Folic Acid!

How romantic... feeding each other folic acid! Honestly though, studies have shown that low sperm count may be attributed to men with low levels of folic acid... so encourage him to eat fortified breakfast cereals, leafy greens, orange juice... or to take a 400-mg. supplement per day. How cute to do it together!

8. Start Taking Vitamin C!

To boost your husband's sperm motility, he must start taking vitamin C. It is recommended that at least 60 mg. per day of vitamin C be added to a man's preconception diet. So toss him an orange, a cantaloupe, or grapefruit… even broccoli (unless his "gas" doesn't need any more help!).

Seriously though, a vitamin C deficiency can cause sperm damage… and even infertility. **C** for yourself how *things* improve!

9. Get Vitamin E Into His Body!

It's all about the sperm, isn't it? Yes! Ah-ha! So to keep them fast, swift, strong, and healthy… it is recommended that men who wish to conceive increase their intake of vitamin E each day. Vitamin E is considered an antioxidant… and antioxidants prevent and/or repair damage to sperm. Plus, it improves circulation… which we like!

Foods high in vitamin E content include nuts, vegetable oils, green leafy vegetables, broccoli (again, at your own risk!), spinach, kiwi, mangos, and fortified cereals. Get him to **E̲at** to keep them swimming!

> **TIDBIT** According to the National Institute of Health, the recommended dietary allowance for vitamin E is 15 milligrams. Supplements list vitamin E in terms of International Units (IU)… 15 milligrams = 22 IU.

10. Get Zinc Into His Body!

Increase your husband's consumption of zinc-filled foods - (here's a plus… oysters, which are rich in zinc, are considered an aphrodisiac as well - ooh-la-la!). Zinc deficiency is associated with low sperm count and lack of sexual potency… but when introduced into the body, zinc actually increases the production of testosterone. Zinc is also reputed to increase sperm count and the production of semen, which, when you're into *baby-making*, is a very, very good thing! Zinc may just be the mightiest MALE mineral of all!

11. Sexually Transmitted Diseases (STDs)

As unlovely as STDs sound… it is crucial that your provider know if your husband has, or has had, a Sexually Transmitted Disease - Gonorrhea, Syphilis, HIV/AIDS, Chlamydia, etc. These are things that you don't want to mess around with, especially if he hasn't received any treatment. These diseases are easily transmitted during sexual encounters, and tragically enough, may lead to male sterility… not to mention female infertility as well, as these transmitted diseases can cause damage to *your* reproductive organs. If necessary, seek treatment immediately.

12. Assess His Occupation

OK… this is not intended to frighten or to alarm you, but to *inform* you. Studies show that male exposure to x-rays, toxic chemicals, paint products, and electromagnetic fields increase the likelihood of babies born prematurely or with birth defects. Again, as with you, sometimes things in life are just the way they are, and it's not possible to change occupations. So, try not to stress or fret about this one; instead, have a healthy discussion with your provider about any possible changes that can be implemented while trying to conceive.

13. Unhealthy Weight!

Just like you, your husband probably doesn't want to hear that he can't or won't be able to conceive a child because of being overweight or underweight (yes, men can be just as stubborn or obsessive as women when it comes to weight issues). His physician should be able to tell your husband if his weight, diet, or eating habits will affect his fertility; but it *is important* for you and your husband to maintain healthy diets… and although you need not give up some of your favorite foods and drinks and snacks, remember that you're trying to prepare your bodies for the healthiest pregnancy, and the healthiest baby.

Our favorite **Your Man** grabber… by far! According to Dr. J. Francois Eid, Director of the Male Sexual Function Unit of New York Presbyterian Hospital… for every thirty-five pounds lost, penis length will *increase* by one inch! Yes… it will *increase* by one inch! Think about it, guys… losing weight will make more of your penis not only more *visible*, but actually more *usable*! Oh… happy day! And if that is not enough to encourage healthy eating habits, studies also show that blood supply is reduced when arteries are lined with cholesterol (from those fatty-food indulgences!), and this lack of blood has a dramatic effect on… you guessed it… the penis!

OLD WIVES' TALE: A man's testicles should be *cool* prior to sex if you want a **daughter**! If a **son** is desired, his testicles should be *warmed* up! How is **up** to you!

14. Excessive Heat or Injuries to "The Boys"!

Sperm production may be decreased by such things as excessive hot tub use, sitting for long periods of time (not the 9am-5pm kind of sitting, but the not-moving-for-24-hours-kind-of-sitting), and tight underwear (maybe you could get him to go without for a bit?)!

Injuries to "The Boys" can wreak all kinds of havoc... from inability to ejaculate, to inability of sperm to reach maturity. It is crucial that your physician be aware of any injuries that your husband may have suffered to the genital area - even as a child (and cyclists, in particular, should make their providers aware of their sport of choice, as extensive cycling has been known to lead to genital injuries). We call this *leaving no stone(s) unturned!*

15. Semen Analysis!

This is one of those things that is generally recommended for couples who are experiencing fertility problems (and often not covered by insurance unless medically indicated), but it could be something that you and your husband just want to have done prior to baby-making.

A Semen Analysis tests for all kinds of things... such as volume of sperm, sperm concentration, sperms' ability to swim, sperm infections, etc. If you feel so inclined, go for it... perhaps you can even provide some provocative photographs of yourself for your husband to bring to the sperm collection session!

~

So... this is about it when it comes to Your Man! As you can see, your husband is just as important as you are in this preconception time! The two of you must work together... and really enjoy this time in your lives. This shouldn't even be considered *work*... this is fun and sexy and exciting and new (for each baby), and should be a very passionate and romantic time in your marriage.

The suggestions we listed should be taken seriously... but have *fun* reading to each other, and getting involved together. Maybe the two of you could join a gym together... or start cooking together... or head to a "vitamin store" to purchase what you may need. Let this be a magnificently healthy *and* sexy *and* relaxing time!

And one more thing! Everyone has a story about her friend's sister's overweight cousin who ate only chocolate ice cream cones and potato chips, drank beer every night, and worked in a environmentally hazardous zone while pregnant, but who had a perfect baby (OK... we're exaggerating a bit)! This could be true, but it's kind of like getting into a rusty old car with little gas, barely enough oil, low tires, no windshield wipers, and thinking (without a doubt) that you'll make it across the country without breaking down. Is it possible? Maybe. It is truly probable? No. Heavy people… skinny people… people who eat junk… people who have never exercised… people who smoke, drink, and abuse illegal substances - they can and do get pregnant every second - but if you want to increase your chances of having healthy babies, all research points to the mental and physical health of the mother and father *prior* to conception. Period!

CHAPTER 3½

Your Hormones - A Brief Primer

NECESSARY INFORMATION FOR WHAT'S TO COME!

Being... is the great explainer.

- *HENRY DAVID THOREAU*

The words testosterone, gonadotropin releasing hormone (GnRH), follicle-stimulating hormone (FSH), luteinizing hormone (LH), estrogen, and progesterone get tossed around in reproductive chat like the ingredients in a salad! Although all ingredients are tasty separately, it's the combination that creates a delicious whole. This is exactly the way your hormones work - maybe not tasty... but they certainly create a delicious whole!

Remember, your hormones are all equally important, and they are your very, very "best friends"...

So no matter how far you venture or roam...
You'll always be accompanied by your friendly hormones!

TESTOSTERONE - your *wild* friend!

Produced by your ovaries and adrenal glands, testosterone is the friend who does-it-all! Fueling your sex drive and energy levels, testosterone steps in to make sure that your clitoris and nipples remain turned to high, and let's face it... perfect for baby-making!

GONADOTROPIN RELEASING HORMONE (GnRH) - your *gossip* friend!

OK... so it does take both sex and brains to make a baby! GnRH, produced in the hypothalamus region of your brain, sends messages to your pituitary gland (also in your brain!), indicating that it's time for ovulation. GnRH gets the process moving forward!

FOLLICLE-STIMULATING HORMONE (FSH) - your *go-to* friend!

FSH springs into action by encouraging the follicle to become mature.

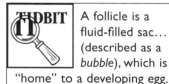

> **TIDBIT** A follicle is a fluid-filled sac... (described as a *bubble*), which is "home" to a developing egg.

LUTEINIZING HORMONE (LH) - your other *go-to* friend!

The LH kicks in by stimulating the mature follicle to release an egg!

ESTROGEN - the friend *you can count on*!

Secreted by your ovaries, estrogen shows up to "primp" your uterus... then she turns her attention to your cervix! She lays a virtual red carpet (well, maybe a *white* carpet), providing a welcoming entrance for baby-making sperm!

> **TIDBIT** Your Luteal Phase begins the day after ovulation, and continues until the day prior to your next period. What is really interesting to note is that this phase is phenomenally consistent among women, lasting 13 - 15 days!

PROGESTERONE - Your *nurturing* friend!

Progesterone, secreted by the corpus luteum (a structure that develops in the ovaries), is the marvelous hormone that prepares your uterus for the imbedding of a fertilized egg. If fertilization does occur, this nurturing hormone helps to strengthen and protect the uterus throughout your pregnancy.

> **TIDBIT** The word progesterone means... literally... *to bear or to carry.*

So... you've met your hormone friends!... always on-duty, always there for you! Ahhh, isn't it absolutely amazing to think about what goes on inside our bodies every day of every month!?

CHAPTER 4

Practice-Makes-Perfect!

While Honey is in Every Flower, no doubt,
It takes a Bee to get the Honey out.
- ARTHUR GUITERMAN

So, how long have you truly given yourself in this preconception time? One month? Three months? Six months? A year?

However long you choose, the beauty and fun and sexiness of this preconception time is in the **Practice-Makes-Perfect!...** and we're talking about the *practice* in knowing your body and the way it works!

This is not just scientific and sound... this is amazing and sexy too! Amazing because you, the woman, the life-giver, the mother-to-be... can *learn* the fertility messages that your body teaches you every day. And sexy because it's the passion, the romance, and your physical body that will bring it all together.

So temperature, mucus, calendars and kits...
Let yourself get into it!

Now, you may read the following fertility message guides and jump into all of them! On the other hand, you may try one or two and say, "Ewww!" to the rest! Really, it's just a personal choice. All we want to do here is give you some options in learning how to predict ovulation, and determine your most fertile days.

If you try any of these methods over a period of time, you will begin to recognize the patterns and rhythms of your own body! Better yet, in the time of *no pressure*, when your confidence is at its peak - **Practice-Will-Make-Perfect** - so, you'll be ready for baby-making when you're ready! Have fun with this chapter... and be open to fascinating possibilities!

We'll start with what we call the "clean and tidy" ones... and save the "down and dirty" ones for last!

BASAL BODY TEMPERATURE (BBT)

Used for decades, BBT works very simply... using a BBT Thermometer (purchased inexpensively at any drug store), you take, and record, your morning body temperature each day. Since thermal changes in your body increase at the on-set of ovulation, your temperature will actually rise - usually between 0.4°F and 0.8°F - *after* you have ovulated. What your body is doing is creating a warm, cozy environment for a potential fertilized egg. The phenomenon of your slight body temperature increase (brought about by the increase of the hormone progesterone) - *at ovulation* - will come to life before your own eyes as you record your temperature each day.

The wisdom in *taking* and *charting* your BBT during your preconception time is that you will begin to know when to anticipate your next ovulation... so when you're ready for your deliciously sexy baby-making sex, you'll approach it with knowledge, confidence, and relaxation!

OVULATION CALENDAR

Still "clean" and pretty easy... the ovulation calendar method predicts ovulation by charting your menstrual cycles over a period of several months. You must keep a very accurate written record of your periods, always circling on your ovulation calendar the first day of each menstrual period. After you have done this for 4 - 6 months... a little 5th grade math kicks in! You identify your shortest menstrual cycle and subtract the number 18 from that number. Then, starting with the date that you circled in your shortest cycle, count forward 10 days. This very date... plus or minus a couple of days... is a prediction of your greatest fertility day! Easy? Yes! Expensive? Try free! Accurate... ? Given the fact that our periods may be affected by so many factors, the ovulation calendar is more a *gauge* of ovulation than a precise indicator.

> **TIDBIT** Two excellent web sites to visit: www.ovulation-calculator.com and www.pregnancy.about.com

If you're into charting and graphing... or just curious... try the BBT *in conjunction* with the ovulation calendar method, perhaps just to see if temperature meets math!

> **TIDBIT** Some women experience what is called Mid-Cycle Spotting... the appearance of a light blood flow during ovulation. If you are one of these women, lucky you! - a built-in ovulation/fertility indicator! This spotting is a result of the slight shedding of the endometrium, those wonderful blood-enriched membranes that have built up in your uterus since your last period!

OVULATION DETECTION KITS

This one involves a little chemistry and a mini-vocabulary lesson! Remember these two terms:

Luteinizing Hormone (LH) - secreted by the pituitary gland, LH is a female hormone needed to regulate ovarian function

LH Surge - the increase in LH, detected in your urine, is indicative of peak fertility!

Now for the chemistry! The good news is that although dozens of these ovulation detection kits are available on the market, their basic principles work the same. The detection of ovulation through these kits involves a chemical reaction that is identified by color changes on supplied testing strips. Simply put, the color changes are directly proportional to your urine's amount of LH at a particular time of the month. What you are looking for is your LH Surge (recognized by color change!), indicative that one of your eggs should be released within 12 - 24 hours, and therefore ovulation should occur!

The slightly bad news is that some of these kits are pricey… so shop around!

Again, your preconception time is a great time to *practice* with your body's fertility messages! You probably don't want your hands shaking… your urine spraying… or to be questioning your attempts to decipher color changes… when your 12 - 24 peak fertility hours become crucial to you!

Remember… **Practice-Makes-Perfect!**

CERVICAL MUCUS

And now for the "down" and… well, not dirty - but kind of messy!

Admittedly or not, we all have cervical mucus. This is a good thing… believe us! Cervical mucus is probably your best guide… in essence, it's your "yellow brick road" in detecting your body's time of ovulation.

So, start looking for cervical mucus… yes, either on your underwear, on toilet paper, and/or on your fingers… immediately after your period stops. At this time, any cervical mucus that you discover will be rather dry... but within a week, you will note marvelous changes! As your body begins to secrete estrogen, the glands around your cervix begin to secrete fluid. Now, at this point, your cervical mucus changes from desert dry to oasis wet (add sticky and whitish)! But... don't let this oasis fool you because there is even more paradise to come!

> **TIDBIT** Have you ever felt "Mittelschmerz"? Translated, this means *middle pain*... a slight ache felt in the lower abdomen during ovulation. Some women feel this each month! Do you?

As ovulation approaches, your body has produced more estrogen, more fluid, and your mucus becomes a virtual *Slip and Slide* - wet, slippery, and stretchable (often described as looking like egg whites - lovely, huh?)! This is when your *lutein* is released... and it is your lutein that allows your ovaries to release an egg. This is the most amazing and sexy miracle because the egg is ready... your mucus is wet and slippery and profuse... your cervix is sperm-inviting and nutritious - all-rolled-into-one... **ovulation**!

Then, if fertilization does not occur, your window of ovulation begins to close, your mucus becomes drier... thicker... and cloudy - a sign of impending menstruation.

But another true miracle of your body is that the cycle begins anew!

Take this journey from "ewww!" to "ahhh!" Become comfortable and relaxed and confident with your cervical mucus indicators during your preconception time. This is a natural and wonderful part of you! And when the time is right... when you and your husband are ready for your delicious baby-making sex... you'll take the slip and slide ride of your life!

CERVICAL POSITION

If you think cervical *mucus* is fun... well, then you'll love cervical *position* as a fertility indicator!

Think of your cervix as the muscle extraordinaire... working beautifully, on its own... without a personal trainer! And as far as *fertility awareness*... examination of the position of your cervix is considered a remarkable fertility predictor! All you need for this is 1 or 2 fingers... OK, now you know what we mean when we say "down and dirty"!

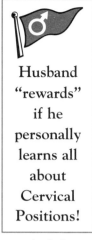

Husband "rewards" if he personally learns all about Cervical Positions!

The beauty of *cervical position* as a fertility indicator is in its simplicity. During infertile periods, such as immediately after menstruation... your cervix is low, quite firm, rather dry, and closed. You (or your husband) can actually *feel* your cervix by gently inserting your finger(s) into your vagina and reaching backwards until you feel the muscle - your cervix!

Still with us!?

As ovulation approaches, the same examination of your cervix will reveal rather dramatic changes. As your estrogen is creating more cervical mucus... your cervix becomes moist, softer, and even more open.

When ovulation occurs... the cervix elevates itself, like a queen at her coronation, and at this point your cervix may even be difficult to reach! Here, your cervix is very soft, completely open, increased in size, and extremely sperm-friendly! Remember... conception cannot take place if the cervix hasn't *risen* to the occasion! *Now* is the time for your "King" to enter the castle if your baby-making time is right!

Following ovulation, the cervix begins its return to a lower... firmer... closed position. It will be easy to reach, but not sperm-friendly! Here, your cervix becomes a servant to no sperm... she's closed for business!

At the risk of sounding repetitive... Practice-Makes-Perfect!

Chances are that you may never have attempted this "search" for your cervix, *and it may take some time to get it right* in order to recognize its changes! Be our guest, or 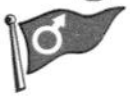 *guests*!

NOTE: *Please... in search of your cervix... always make sure that fingers are thoroughly washed before (and after) you go on in!*

~

It's so funny that in our technically advanced world, we think nothing of sending and receiving telephone messages, cell phone messages, e-mail messages; we check our banking, we make our reservations, we even purchase homes and cars online. But when it comes to receiving our own *body's* messages, in the greatest miracle of all - ovulation - many of us are so busy questioning the "what ifs" (what if I can't get pregnant? what if it takes years? what if there's something wrong?) that we don't recognize the most natural gifts of all.

This is precisely why we have said to take your *preconception time* to get to know your body and its messages... which will lead to confidence, relaxation, and deliciously sexy sex at any time of the month, but most particularly when you are ready for baby-making!

Take this preconception time to recognize that your body, like clockwork, sends you direct "c-mail" (cervix mail!) messages each and every month!

Receive them and reply!

Practice-Makes-Perfect!

CHAPTER 5

Conception

A journey of a thousand miles must begin
with a single step.
- *CHINESE PROVERB*

Believe it or not, many, many women (and even more men!) have only a vague idea, or no idea at all, about what occurs at the moment of conception. The hope of that very moment is probably why you are reading this book... why you are so excited about preparing your bodies for that moment... and why, let's be honest, we're all here to talk about it! So here's a crash course for those of you who need it (even us!):

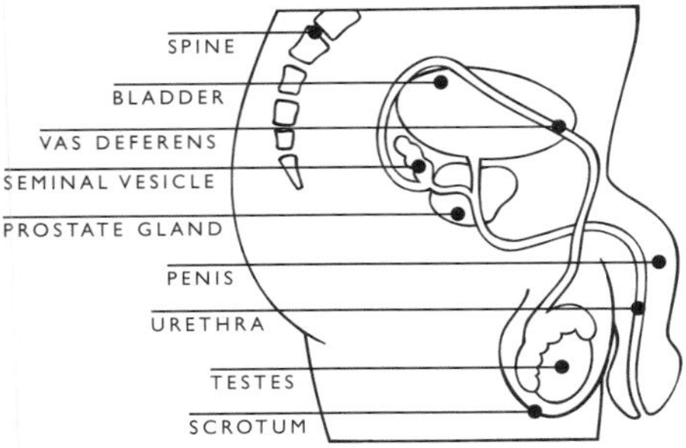

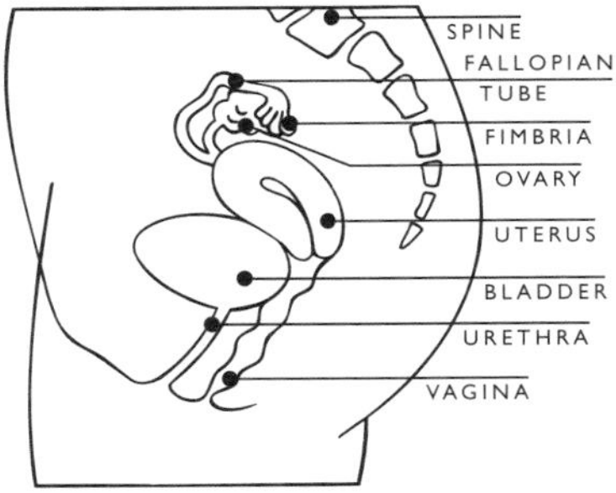

Women have 2 ovaries... 2 fallopian tubes... 1 uterus... 1 cervix... and 1 vagina (well... hopefully)! Each month, on approximately Day 14 of your menstrual cycle (counting Day 1 as the *first* day of your last period), an egg (ovum) is released from one ovary into its corresponding fallopian tube. At this point, your hormones kick in and help contract the egg toward the mother ship, the uterus. Some women get crampy and actually *feel* the contractions as the egg starts its journey!

Men have a penis… and for now, that's all you need to know!...(but for those who *absolutely* need to know more, see the TidBIG on page 57)!

The most interesting thing about any eventual 7-pound (or so) baby is that everything starts off microscopically. We mean… so microscopically that the average mature egg that a woman releases is (get this!) approximately 1/175 inch in diameter, and weighs approximately 1/20 of a millionth of an ounce! We're talking *tiny* - unable to be seen by the naked eye… so the fact that some women *feel* this egg starting on its journey is miraculous, to say the least.

And if you think the egg is tiny, it is downright *enormous* compared to the (dare we say, minuscule!) male sperm cell comprised of:

1) **an oval-shaped head,** which contains the most important structure in egg fertilization and development;
2) **connecting middle piece,** which helps the little guy swim properly; and
3) **a whip-like tail,** which measures approximately 1/500 inch in length, and really puts the pedal to the metal!

And weight? Why is it that weight is always in issue!? It takes about 90,000 sperm cells to equal the weight of just one egg! Yes… 90,000!

So now that you have some mental images of the egg and the sperm cells, let's talk about sex!

During your deliciously sexy sex, the sperm are sent swimming (ejaculation) in a race… get this… with up to three-hundred million competitors (want to make your husband feel important tonight? Share that "three-hundred million" little tidbit with him about his "Boys")! And for a little more information about him, the male carries both the X and Y chromosomes, and single-handedly (or single-"spermedly"!) determines the sex of your baby. And to make him feel *even more virile* tonight, share with him the news that the ejaculated three-hundred million sperm are but a drop in the bucket for him, as he is able to produce hundreds of millions more tomorrow... and if he remains healthy, each day for the rest of his life! Va... va... va-voom!

OK... back to the sperm! Now that the sperm have entered the cervix, they are in the race of their lives to be the ONE - emphasize ONE - that reaches the "come and get me" egg waiting in the fallopian tube... but (of course!), these "Boys" must rely on a little help from the woman! Right at the time of ovulation... the vagina, the cervix, the uterus, and the fallopian tubes change from an acidic (kills sperm) to an alkaline (loves sperm) environment. This alkaline environment, as one would expect, is heavenly to sperm!

At the cervix, the competing sperm are also met with welcoming mucus... only, however, when the woman is ovulating - and again, this helps as many sperm as possible survive. The heartiest of the still-swimming-competitors enter the uterus, where some of the less fortunate ones (we'll try not to call them underachievers!) swim into the wrong fallopian tube and are lost.

At this point, it's the survival of the fittest! As the egg is being contracted downward through the fallopian tube toward the uterus, the sperm are swimming upward through the uterus toward the egg. It is this approximate *5-inch race* that truly separates the *Man* from the *Boys*, for of the now hundreds of sperm that arrive at the site of the egg, only ONE wins... and that winner immediately stakes its claim.

This is the very moment of conception!

What happens next is both scientific and miraculous! The now fertilized egg's cells multiply into a ball of cells, and within (usually) 3-4 days, travels to the cozy, comfortable, and welcoming uterus. It then burrows itself into the uterine wall, which becomes its comfy home for the next nine (or so) months.

For the purposes of this book, we'll stop here, as there are zillions of resources that bring you from this moment right through birth. And as soon as you do conceive, it will absolutely warm your heart to read about that exciting time in your life - your pregnancy!

> **TIDBIT** This is when you will come to love the words "Chorionic Gonadotropin (hCG)". Although this sounds like something you may purchase at an auto repair shop, it is actually the wonderful hormone that your body produces once your fertilized egg has embedded itself into your uterine wall! The presence of hCG will give you 2 lines on a pregnancy test indicator… showing that, yes... you are pregnant!

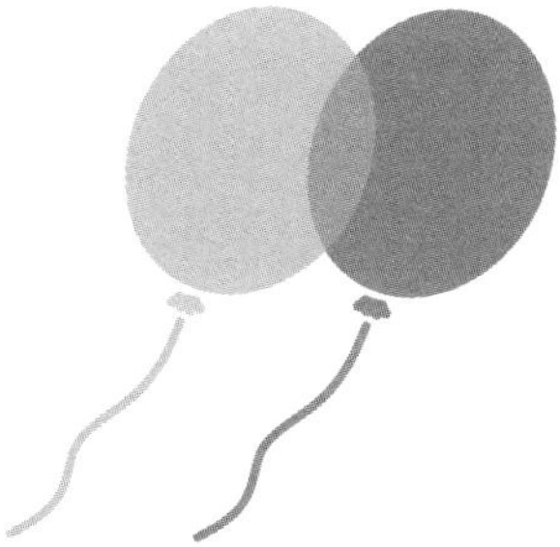

PART TWO

The Wings

The soul is the voice of the body's interest.
-GEORGE SANTAYANA

"A mystical experience is the awareness of a Presence and the consciousness of a Beyond." What could be more holy, mystical, and miraculous in the mosaic of the universe than you and your husband bringing a child into this world!? Even though you exist in the here and now - the *Present* - you are thinking of a *Beyond*... which has been shaped by the *Past*!

Until now, you have been reading medical and scientific information and facts about healthy preconception, but from here on in you will be immersed in natural, wonderful, and sometimes universal beliefs surrounding preconception. **PART II** of this book, what we call **THE WINGS**, is intended to give you freedom and fun and flights of fancy in your journey to becoming a parent.

You will gain wisdom in enhancing your fertility through the use of such wonders as foods and drinks, aphrodisiacs, aromas, herbs, amulets, dance and music, and, of course... delicious sex! You may even begin to look at yourself, your husband, and your future baby(ies) as marvelous and miraculous pieces of the universe, and recognize the idea that there are so many levels to explore in fertility knowledge - such as the fertility cycle reflecting the 29-day moon cycle... the aspects of color... fertility gems and stones... the power of prayer, blessings, rituals, journaling - and touches of magic!

So whether you just *enjoy* the myths and folklore and cultural traditions coming from different corners of the universe... or you feel that the traditions may *enhance* your body, mind, and spirit in preparation for conception… or you absolutely *embrace* these traditions as a way to become a piece of the universe… or you become truly *ecstatic* with the revelations and do everything possible at your fingertips - whether you are cautious or casual or carefree…

Indulge! Indulge! Indulge!

Spread your Wings!

CHAPTER 6

Food Aphrodisiacs

Men are like bagpipes... nothing comes from them unless they're full.

-SCOTTISH PROVERB

Aphrodisiacs (named for Aphrodite, the ancient Greek Goddess of sensual love) arouse sexual desires and passions. It may be the vitamins, the minerals, or the nutrients that increase blood flow to our genital areas - but who cares why!? For your purposes, sexual desire leads to delicious sex, delicious sex leads to incredible warmth and relaxation, and incredible relaxation of your body will help lead to a beautiful conception, a magnificent pregnancy, and a healthy baby!

Aphrodisiacs are not mysterious, secretive, or naughty oils and gels that you purchase from the internet! Aphrodisiacs are fabulous, fun, often common-yet-wonderful foods and scents and spices and herbs that we consume every single day. The beauty of aphrodisiacs for deliciously sexy baby-making is that they enhance your sexual desire and harness the astonishing powers that aphrodisiacs bring to fertility!

Baby-making needs to be a relaxing, sexy, wonderful time.

You are meant to and deserve to feel good, look good, possess confidence, be relaxed, and fully enjoy pleasure. All of the foods on our **SHOPPING LIST** bring these gifts to you, to your husband, and to your babies. Even the ancients knew that healthy foods and great sex - and the union of male and female energies - is what creates fertilization of not only the people, but the land, and the entire world as well!

So, if you're going to know *what* to eat, you may as well know *why it works*! There is nothing mysterious here. In fact, it is all quite simple. Keep these secrets to yourself… or share them at your will… the mini "physiology" lesson is as follows:

> *Even though* ***estrogen*** *is considered a "female" hormone, and* ***testosterone*** *is considered a "male" hormone, it is* ***testosterone*** *that fuels sexual arousal in* ***both men and women****. Once sexually stimulated, a testosterone kick from aphrodisical foods sends wonderful signals from the brain, through the nervous system, to yes… the pelvic region. Ah-ha! This is what we like! There, blood vessels open and the blood takes a mad rush to the erectile tissues - in both men and women… and we all know what happens next!*

SO LET'S START WITH FOOD! A romantic interlude seems always to involve food! Our favorite is a nice homemade meal with romantic candlelight. There's nothing like eating at home - to dress in any way you desire (which could be dangerous!), with your favorite music… maybe even a crackling fire… just the two of you. Just *thinking* about it could get you going!

So getting into a sensuous mood…
May simply be about the foods!

Grab your **SHOPPING LIST** and run… run… run… to your market. Tonight, both of you are in for a treat!

Shopping List

This Shopping List is available for your shopping convenience - see Appendix, page 203!

APPETIZERS

Always the start of something good!

ARTICHOKES

Any way you care to prepare them, artichokes have been known to increase jumbo (yee-haa!) blood flow to the genitals! Yum-yum-yummy! Containing lusty vitamins and minerals such as C, B6, zinc, folic acid, and potassium, artichokes have been enjoyed and "employed" for centuries! As a matter of fact, some 16th century "prudes" forbade women the pleasure of eating artichokes, as artichokes were thought to enhance sexual power… but the men were allowed to have their fill! Hmmm! You may be inclined to *make up* for all those years of denial!

CAVIAR

Splurge ladies! Caviar may be one of the most expensive foods you may ever purchase (especially caviar from the Beluga sturgeon, which takes about twenty years to mature before producing eggs!), but caviar dramatically (yes, *dramatically*) increases strong erections. Caviar is very low in calories, but very rich in proteins and those all-important omega-3 fatty acids. So

> **TIDBIT** According to Ellen and Michael Albertson, authors of ***Temptations***, the Greeks started their version of a cocktail party (otherwise known as an "orgy") by passing around hors d'oeuvres that consisted of caviar, oysters, and (hmm…?) roasted grasshoppers!

don't let the fact that caviar is really fish eggs turn you off… on the contrary, you'll be *on* all night long!

> **TIDBIT** According to Adelheid Ohlig, author of ***Luna Yoga…*** highly recommended fertility-increasing foods for both men and women include sour milk products such as yogurt, buttermilk, kefir, whey, curds, quark, cottage cheese, and ricotta… but keep in mind that non-pasteurized cheeses may contain harmful bacteria and should be avoided if you become pregnant.

CHEESE

Ahhh… cheese! With crackers, in dips, or just plain - with its combination of protein and calcium, cheeses are easy sexual energizers to serve and to eat. So slice, dice, grate, melt, and serve… you just gotta love cheese!

ENDIVE

Think cool and crisp! Eat it by itself, or add this curly, leafy, vitamin A-enriched lettuce* variety to your favorite salad. Either way, you'll toss the lust factor *up* a notch!

**Not to scare you… sorry, salad lovers - but lettuce, consumed in large amounts, is believed by some dietitians to lead to sterility in both men and women; and excessive ingestion of vitamin A has been associated with birth defects.*

> **TIDBIT** And just so you know why vitamin A is so important… it is required for normal reproductive functioning, with great influence on the development of sperm, ovaries, and placenta! And once pregnant… keep eating, as vitamin A aids in normal development of the embryo and fetus!

GUACAMOLE

Olé! Or if you prefer… Oh-lay! This green dish, comprised of avocados, chilis, onions, and tomatoes, is a wonderfully stimulating romantic-evening dip to purchase or whip up together! How **"hot"** are you feeling? This mixture, rich in vitamin E (hold on ladies!), increases sperm production, promotes blood flow, and leads to stronger erections. Imagine this with *oysters*! Read on…

OYSTERS

If you and your husband are seafood lovers... this may be all you need! Rich in zinc (remember its importance from **Your Man** chapter?), oysters send testosterone-sperm-producing-male-hormones through the roof! So scrape yourself off the ceiling! But honestly, the real skinny is quite remarkable... oysters are considered "cupid's arrow"! They contain a perfect combination of protein, complex sugars, minerals, and irons to feed *both* the male and female's lust, passion, and desire. Don't shy away from these seductive edibles... grab a cookbook, as there are dozens of ways to enjoy them!

MAIN DISHES

The "main" attractions!

BEEF

A nice juicy steak - many a man's dream (of course, served by you... naked)! Rich in zinc and protein, red meat enhances the sexual vitality hormones that get you going... and, in moderate amounts, beef increases much needed concentration - yeah, baby! Choose the leaner cuts, though... just keep thinking: smaller beef portions = additional weight control = larger penis (see page 64)!

> **TIDBIT** Poultry! Although poultry isn't known for its aphrodisical qualities, you can turn up its heat with unlimited varieties of aphrodisiac herbs (pages 96 - 97), spices (pages 97 - 99), and sauces with which to *dress* your poultry. Remember that *dressing* your poultry may just be the way to *undress* the two of you... and poultry's power-packed-protein is sure to *rev* up your engines as well!

OLD WIVES' TALE: If you want a **boy**... make sure that both you and your husband eat lots of meat!

SEAFOOD

The guy at the fish market may just become your new best friend! The Hebrew word for fish - *nun* - means *to sprout or put forth*, referring to the conceiving or bearing of children! Whatever your preference - salmon, scallops, lobster, shrimp, swordfish, mussels, octopus, squid, conch, anchovies, sardines, mackerel, tuna, shark, snails, even eel...! - fish contains omega-3 fatty acids, zinc, protein, phosphorous, and iodine - all ingredients that strengthen sexual vitality. ♂ Fish is also loaded with magnesium, which seemingly and magically allows more blood flow to the penis! So walk, run, swim if you must - just get some seafood into your *main* meals!

TIDBIT Keep in mind that most physicians recommend avoiding cooked shark, tuna, swordfish, king mackerel, and all raw fish if conception is your *immediate aim*, or if you are *already pregnant*... as these are reputed to not only contain absorbed toxins and mercury, but they add risks of food-borne illnesses as well.

A WORD TO THE WISE:

Although disputed by the farmed salmon industry, findings indicate that farmed salmon may contain higher levels of Polychlorinated Biphenyls (PCBs - industrial by-products linked to cancer and fetal brain development) than those found in ocean salmon... but the United States Food and Drug Administration (FDA) is sticking by its advice that Americans should consume salmon, and fish, as part of a healthy diet.

HOT DOGS

No nutritional or aphrodisical qualities what-so-ever! Just plain fun to watch each other eat!

VEGETABLES

You'll be glad you got hooked on these "treats" early on (if your Mom only knew)!

ASPARAGUS

Take a quick peek at these tall stalks… not only rich in vitamin E (keeps him going all-night-long), but actually resemble what we'll call "The Phallic Giant"!

> **TIDBIT** Vitamins B, C, and E in your husband's diet are important for healthy sperm and sperm count! Just think…
> **B**, **C**, and **E** =
> **Big Constant Erections!**

CARROTS

Another "Giant" shape, and literally packed with vitamins A, C, and E, carrots are known to increase lust, love, fertility, and especially male potency! And we always thought carrots were just good for your eyes!

OLD WIVES' TALE: If you want a **girl**, make sure that both you and your husband eat lots of fish and vegetables!

CELERY

Another "Giant" in the aphrodisiac world! This seemingly unassuming little vegetable is loaded with vitamin C, potassium, calcium, and iron… and more importantly, for your needs - celery contains the male sex hormone androsterone! With the combination of all these "good boys"… he will not be able to keep his hands off of you! Honestly… who would have thought that all these goodies could be packed into that simple, smooth, slender stalk!? Oh, my!

CHILI PEPPERS

Sweet and hot… well, very *sweaty* and hot… we're sure you'll want the *sweating* to continue even after you eat (*dinner*, that is!).

Throughout all history and across multiple cultures, people have used chili peppers - loaded with vitamins A, C, and E - to stimulate endorphin production, which results in incredibly sustained energy. And... we're sure you know by now that incredibly sustained energy continues right into the bedroom!

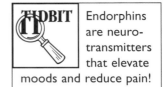

> **TIDBIT** Endorphins are neurotransmitters that elevate moods and reduce pain!

CUCUMBERS

Ooohhh baby! This is a *big one* (pun intended!) in the aphrodisiac world! This "Giant", filled with zinc and vitamins A and C, will not only put you in the mood, but its aroma has been known to increase vaginal flow. Seriously, we're not kidding here! No wonder it's considered a fertility and potency enhancer! Hmmm... and we're wondering why there are now so many cucumber-based soaps and lotions and beauty products!?

MUSHROOMS

And yet another "Giant" in the vegetable kingdom! Mushrooms, packed with magnesium, potassium, and phosphorus, are often associated with sexual potency and fertility. In fact, the mushroom is the symbol of re-birth in China. So... take it from us - sauté them, grill them, or *use* them raw... just eat 'em!

ONIONS

Load up on these lusty little hot devils! Your tears will be for passion and joy! Containing vitamin C, folic acid, and potassium... onions are known worldwide and across all cultures as invigorating... blood-pumping... sperm-increasing fare. Dare eat them raw!?... if *both* of you indulge, of course!

RADISHES

Filled with excellent sources of vitamin C, folic acid, potassium, and magnesium… this purplish-red veggie is a natural lust-inducer. Make sure that these seductive little goodies find their way to your mouths!

TOMATOES

Whether you consider the tomato a fruit or a vegetable… who cares! Its red color inspires passion and love… and its luscious juices get your own juices pumping! Loaded with vitamin C… you may want to head right to the bedroom after eating!

ZUCCHINI

This "Giant" relies on its shape alone! Just the seductiveness of the word and shape could drive you crazy! Steam it… grill it… fry it! Filled with vitamin C… eat it any way you desire, just as long as you get it down!

ON THE SIDE

For some added pleasure!

RICE

You may be interested to know that rice is tossed at newly married couples as a fertility charm, for it is known in many cultures as the "staff of life"… but for your baby-making purposes, you will want to spice up your rice dishes and recipes with any number of aphrodisiac herbs and/or spices (see pages 96 - 99) in order to *fully* appreciate the *powers* of rice!

SWEET POTATOES

Sweet potatoes, rich in vitamins B and C, are reputed to increase sexual lust and desire. So do yourself a favor… serve them more often than just with your Thanksgiving meal! Go ahead... be "sweet" *and* naughty with this one all year long!

HERBS

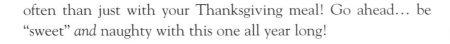

Dash away to another world!

A WORD TO THE WISE:

According to Adelheid Ohlig, author of **Luna Yoga**, sprouts from any beans - including alfalfa sprouts, mung bean sprouts, and lentil sprouts - *inhibit* fertility! This was first observed in animals grazing on such plants.

BASIL

Basil is known to rev up your sex drive and to boost fertility! Loaded with vitamins A, B6, and C, folic acid, calcium, iron, magnesium, and zinc... basil is not just for eating! As a touch of magic, fresh basil leaves rubbed against your skin act as nature's aphrodisiac. Hmmm... do the initials **BBT** actually stand for ***Basil* Body Temperature**!?

CAPERS

The unopened green flower buds of the "cappars spinoso" bush, capers range in size from... well, very tiny to very small! Low in sodium, capers invigorate us with vitamins A, C, and E, folic acid, iron, and magnesium! A lust-inducing food, capers are reputed to cure impotency in men! Hmmm... is it any surprise that "caper" also means *to dance, frolic, leap, or play*!?

DILL

A very good source of calcium, iron, magnesium, zinc, and vitamin C, dill is a lust-inducer! But don't just cook with dill... as a touch of magic, toss dill into your bath, as the scent will make you absolutely irresistible to your husband. Maybe he'll jump in and join you! Think **dill**-icious!

GARLIC

This one may surprise you with its "stanking" reputation… but, in fact, garlic has historically been known as a lust and passion-inducer. Why? Garlic is a wonderful source of vitamins B6 and C, calcium, and phosphorus! Stir up your sexual desires by adding this hot little number to your recipes! Cut it. Grate it. Dice it. Chop it. Light up your night with this bulb!

> **TIDBIT** It has been noted that garlic works along the same lines as Viagra!

PARSLEY

Like many herbs, parsley is loaded with vitamins A and C, calcium, phosphorus, magnesium, iron, and potassium, and is known for its powers of fertility… so "Dash away! Dash away! Dash away, all!" And as a touch of magic, include parsley… mixed with the nuts and seeds of your choice… in a daily fertility-stimulating side dish!

SPICES

Let's turn it up a notch!

CINNAMON

Huge! Huge! Huge! A very good source of vitamin C, calcium, and iron… cinnamon is a lust-inducing spice that fights fatigue! Nobody wants to be tired during sex, so sprinkle liberally! Come on, ladies… sprinkle some cinnamon on your (or his) "buns"!

CLOVES

A deliciously fragrant spice, loaded with vitamin C, iron, calcium and magnesium… cloves lustfully attract your lover! Add henever possible (and appropriate)! Cloves... sure troves! OK, cloves are considered a ant because they are shaped like tiny penises!

GINGER

Ginger, filled with vitamin C, potassium, and phosphorus... and known for its pungent quality... fires *up* the body in all the right ways. Be adventurous... try this at breakfast, lunch, *and* dinner! Ginger has a reputation of driving women wild, and we certainly like that!

NUTMEG

Nutmeg is not only low in sodium and cholesterol, but it is a great fiber source as well. Like ginger, nutmeg fires *up* the body, and is known to dramatically prolong sexual performance. Don't just top your eggnog with nutmeg! Bake with it... sprinkle it... and really *cook* with it! Supposedly... mixing nutmeg with honey and a half-boiled egg (and eaten one hour prior to sex) makes a sex tonic that prolongs performance!

PEPPER (Black, Green, and White)

Pepper contains all of the "hotties"... vitamin C, calcium, magnesium, iron, and potassium... and is known to make your husband that much *hotter* by strengthening nerves and circulation! This increased stamina certainly helps in the you-know-what department!

SAFFRON

Why does the word *Hallelujah!* come to mind when saffron is mentioned!? Containing vitamins B6 and C, iron, and magnesium, and at one time offered to fertility Goddess Astoreth,

> **TIDBIT** Astoreth was especially revered as a Goddess who brought special blessings to the *family,* and who helped people realize their dreams.

saffron imitates sex hormones and heightens sensitivity - you know where - to create ecstasy! After a night of adding this big-girl to your culinary delights, you just may want to name your next baby Saffron (if it's a girl, of course)!

FRUITS

Juicy and delicious!

APPLES

> **TIDBIT** Apples... Apples...! Because of the many seeds that an apple contains, in some cultures apples are known as fertility enhancers - hence the term "Love Apples"!

If an apple a day keeps the doctor away, let's hope your husband / wife isn't a doctor! Apples, which are filled to the brim with vitamins A and C, folic acid, and potassium, have been the subject of myths, legends, and fairy tales for centuries... and for good reason! Apples arouse sexual desire... plain and simple. So eat them any way you can... fresh, dried, cooked, baked - they will forever live in the land of erotic fantasy. Delight in them! And as a touch of magic, bake the spice *cardamom* into your apple pie to *further* excite sexual passion... believe us, it works!

APRICOTS

The juices alone are symbols of sexuality! Very rich in vitamin C... go on, feed each other!

BANANAS

Come on, ladies... need we say more!? Just look at one... hold one... and open your mouth to take a bite - what comes to mind!? Or is that just us? OK... we'll indulge you a bit! Bananas are rich in vitamin B and potassium, known ingredients to increase fertility and cure impotency! Oh, it *isn't* just us!?

DATES

Not just something you do on Saturday nights! These little treats (rich in both protein and fat, as well as vitamins A, B, and C, calcium, and iron) pack a double whammy - they increase fertility *and* sexual potency. The fruit of the date palm tree, dates symbolize fertility because of the large number of dates produced by each tree. Eat your dates (we're not going there!) to increase fertility, and as a touch of magic... ask your husband to carry the nut (not going there either!) to increase sexual potency! Guess you'd better stock up on dates, huh!?

FIG

The fig - a huge fertility "Giant" - was honored by the Greeks, Hindus, Romans, and Egyptians as an exquisitely sexually-charged fruit for both the male and female! Containing potassium, calcium, and iron, as well as high in fiber, fresh figs are known to cure impotency and infertility in men! It is such a powerful force... that for centuries women have carried figs as symbols of fertility. How's that for a touch of magic!

GRAPES

Red or green - fresh grapes are packed with vitamins A, B6, and C, as well as folic acid. Actually, grapes are pretty simple... fermented, they are made into wines, and wine is considered the most romantic of beverages! And, grapes are considered a fertility enhancer. As a touch of magic, grab your paint brushes, for legend has it that to ensure fertility, pictures of grapes should be painted, sketched, or stenciled on (or in) your home, or along garden walls!

MANGOES

Packed with vitamins A and C, mangoes enhance fertility as well as allow for a delicious oral encounter! In India, the mango tree is considered a sacred symbol of love... and as a touch of magic, some believe that the mango tree has the power to grant wishes!

MELONS

Sexy, ripe, juicy, and nutritious... just like the nature of a woman! Filled with vitamins A and C, and potassium, yield to the pleasures of melons! Yield all the way!

OLIVES

Olives... like men... either small, medium, large, extra-large, jumbo, colossal, super colossal, black, or green (if they're from another planet)! Olives are known for their powers of fertility, lust, and potency because of their incredible vitamin A content - and we're talking *sexual* potency! Consider this touch of cultural magic... Athenian brides were known to wear olive leaf crowns to guarantee fertility!

ORANGES

Fragrant and wet, and just teeming with vitamins A and C, calcium, and iron, oranges provoke feelings of love! In ancient times, oranges were even offered as gifts to newly married couples in order to increase their fertility. Oranges are also reputed to be a symbol of fruitfulness and fertility because the tree is considered *ever*green, and *ever-bearing* of fruits and flowers. Go ahead... suck on a navel!

PAPAYAS

Think juicy. Think large. You still there? Think feeding one another... piece by piece... this fleshy tropical fruit! And if that's not enough, consider that the papaya is an excellent source of vitamin C and folic acid, and known to increase lustful feelings! The papaya may make your husband *a papa* for *ya*!

PEACHES

Pulpy... sweet... juicy... and magical! Peaches, naturally packed with vitamins A and C, and potassium, are not only known for their fertility powers, but they are sexy-sexy-sexy to eat! As a touch of magic... in some cultures the branches of peach trees are used as magical wands. Why not bring a branch into your bedroom! And as a side note, an interesting fact about the peach is that in both China and Japan, the peach is revered as a fertility symbol... and peach blossoms are often worn or carried by brides to enhance fertility!

> **TIDBIT** According to the United States Department of Health and Human Services... and the National Cancer Institute... men should be encouraged to "shoot for nine" - by consuming **nine servings** of fruits and vegetables each day! A medium piece of fruit, or 6 oz. of 100% fruit juice, is considered one ideal serving!

PEARS

Fleshy and shapely (like a woman!) and richly flavored... the pear is known to increase sexual arousal! Maybe it's the potassium, the iron, or the calcium! Maybe it's the way you must open your mouth wide enough to get a good solid bite... until the juices flow! Maybe you should just indulge!

STRAWBERRIES

The red, juicy strawberry can evoke sensually stimulating sex! As an appetizer, snack, or dessert... this luscious and nutritious fruit is known for its lustfully stimulating vita-

> **TIDBIT** The strawberry is a member of the Rose Family... the most love and lust-inducing of all flowers!

min C, folic acid, and potassium content… and for its "get you in the mood" powers. As a touch of magic, carry the leaves of the strawberry for luck.

CONDIMENTS

Did you think we were about to say something else!?

HONEY

Besides *imagining* what you could do with honey, the good news is - indulge! Honey is known as a virility enhancer. Why? The glucose in honey is absorbed quickly by the body to *provide* immediate energy… and wait!… there's more! The fructose in honey is absorbed slowly enough to *sustain* that energy! As a matter of fact, in a recent study out of London, the ancient alcoholic beverage *honey mead* (a mixture of fermented honey and water) was put to the sex test. Results? Pretty much the same increased sex drive as "reported" in ancient times (see **Mead**, pages 107)!

> **TIDBIT** Cupid is said to have dipped his arrows in honey in order to sweeten the hearts of lovers.

MUSTARD

Mustard seed, aided by its calcium, iron, magnesium, and protein content, increases fertility in women by enhancing sex hormones! So spread mustard on your favorite foods… and on your favorite places!

> **TIDBIT** Much has been written about the mustard seed… from its power as an antidote for poisonous insect bites, to its ability to strengthen the heart and provide blood flow to those all-important places!

DESSERTS

And count yourself a dessert too!

OLD WIVES' TALE: If you want a **girl**... allow your chocolate cravings to overtake you!

CHOCOLATE

Oh, yes!... this "dangerous" little pleasure, chocolate is loaded with the stimulant Phenylethylamine (PEA - an endogenous neuroamine/antidepressant), and therefore chocolate does it all... from increasing energy, to exciting excitement, to stimulating sexual arousal and pleasure! Perhaps chocolate should just be the entire meal!? And as a touch of magic, some believe that green M&Ms in particular are lusty little aphrodisiacs. Hey... *green* does mean *go*!

TIDBIT Ever wonder why women are the ones who crave chocolate? Studies suggest that women are more affected by the "magic" of Phenylethylamine. Who cares if we can't pronounce it!?... as long as it makes us feel really, really, really happy!

ECLAIRS

Have you ever seen an éclair? Held one? Eaten one? The shape... the custard... we're blushing just mentioning it! OK... not really! But as far back as the Middle Ages, Liebesknochen (translated - "bone of love"), otherwise known as éclairs, were baked and eaten and enjoyed as part of *fertility* customs. Wonder why? Yumma! Yumma!

♂ LICORICE (Black only!)

Licorice!? Honestly... when was the last time you even thought of licorice? But this long "bad boy" is known to enhance erectile function! And while feeding it to your husband... as *hard* as it may be to believe, consider that the combined aromas of licorice and cucumber are reputed to *increase vaginal blood flow* as well. So stock *up* on both licorice* and cucumbers... for your dessert pleasures!

TIDBIT The word licorice means *sweet root* (ooh... la... la)! Even the ancient Hindus used licorice (mixed with milk and sugar) to increase sexual prowess. But, in our opinion, the Irish have the best name for licorice - "Maiden Milis" - translated, this means *sugar stick*!

Studies indicate that* ***excessive* *licorice ingestion may cause electrolyte imbalance and high blood pressure.*

PUMPKIN PIE

The scent of any home-cooked pie may send your husband "coming" (pun intended)... but pumpkin pie, abundant in phosphorus, is known to increase penile blood flow by up to 40%! And according to Dr. Alan Hirsch, at the Smell and Taste Treatment and Research Foundation in Chicago, "The combination of pumpkin pie *and lavender* boosts penile blood flow" as well. According to Dr. Hirsch, these smells "may trigger feelings of comfort, security and nostalgia, which can lower anxiety, a major mood breaker." Just be prepared for neighbors' inquiries as to the constantly wafting pumpkin pie aromas coming from your home all year long!

VANILLA

Like its lusty friend chocolate, vanilla is known to attract the opposite sex. Vanilla's *scent* in particular not only calms and relaxes, but it also acts as a powerful and mysterious erotic sex enhancer. Experiment with your vanilla... ice cream cones (oh, my!), candies, smoothies, vanilla extract baths, candles, or all of the above... simultaneously!

TIDBIT The word vanilla is derived from the Latin word *vagina* - yes... vagina!

LATE NIGHT SNACKS

In the special case that you're "up" late!

SEEDS AND NUTS (all varieties!)

Well, now... how could we not include this category... as nuts and seeds are known as incredible fertility inducers! Nature's perfect foods, nuts and seeds are loaded with perfectly proportioned fatty acids, vitamin E, zinc, protein, and complex carbohydrates - all nutrients that will rock your world! These little babies can be carried anywhere and eaten at any time - the perfect aphrodisiac! And they certainly knew what they were doing in Germany, as at one time the almond cookie Mandelcher was designed and baked to resemble and represent testicles (of course!)... and eaten as a symbol of masculine virility! Please pass the cookies!

> **TIDBIT** You must crack the nuts before you can eat the kernal.
> - IRISH PROVERB

Some of our favorite nuts and seeds include:

Caraway - bake caraway into cakes, breads, and cookies to induce lust!

Chestnut - known as a great lust-inducer... feed chestnuts to your lover, perhaps over an open fire?

Hazelnut - when consumed, hazelnuts have been known to increase fertility!

Pumpkin - remember the increased penile blood flow (see Pumpkin Pie, page 105)?

Sesame - when consumed, sesame seeds also act as lust-inducers!

Sunflower - eat sunflower seeds *if* and *when* you wish to conceive!

BEVERAGES

Wet, warming, and wonderful!

**Although you have been advised to refrain from all alcoholic beverages while preparing to conceive, you may not yet be actively preparing! You know yourself if it's safe to drink an alcoholic beverage or two. It truly depends upon where you are in this preconception time. Just be smart... careful... and responsible!*

BEER*

Honestly... since you're getting ready for conception, keep in mind that alcohol increases blood flow *only* when consumed in moderation - that's one or two drinks. Sorry guys, but it's either "The Giant" comes out to play or "The Giant" goes to sleep!

CHAMPAGNE*

A bit of champagne often decreases inhibitions, and may even get you further into the mood for delicious sex! Don't forget... for even more sexual stimulation, add some strawberries... or a vanilla bean or two... to your champagne toast! Trust us!

LEMON TEA / LEMONADE

Simply put, lemon tea and lemonade increase (you guessed it!) lust and sex drive! Maybe it's the vitamin C kicking in!? Whether hot or cold... you'll get the same *hot* results!

♂ MEAD

Make sure *your* "Honey" reads this! Already mentioned in our condiment section under **Honey**, Mead is a fermented mixture of honey and water and spices, rich in the essential blood-pumping vitamin B complex. How about visiting a web site such as http://www.rabbitsfootmeadery.com for recipes, purchasing information, and the fun that will follow!

MILK

Yes… with its vitamins A and D, and calcium, milk *does do a body good*! Especially associated with motherhood - milk should be a beverage of choice. And since the fat content in milk can now be so greatly reduced, there is simply no excuse to avoid this rich gift of nature! So go on… do your body good… and drink up!

PEPPERMINT TEA

Iced or hot! In ancient times, peppermint tea was believed to increase virility and stimulate passion, and was referred to as "Aphrodite's Crown"! And Aphrodite certainly knew what she was doing, since peppermint is abundant in vitamins A and C, folic acid, calcium, iron, zinc, magnesium, and phosphorus! Brew *up* some peppermint tea for both of you! Take a *hint*… as to what you can do with pepper*mint*!

SAKE*

Derived from rice, sake is a symbol of fertility in many cultures… and revered for its rice derivation, sake is used in many cultural and holiday celebrations. Most sacred and magical, offer a toast to your lover! Say it with sake!

SMOOTHIES

A great alternative to alcohol, gather your favorite aphrodisical fruits and/or spices and watch these ingredients blend into seductive colors and textures and aromas. Experiment! Drink up!

TEQUILA*

Known to increase sexual desire, just remember that *too* much tequila may make your memory of the delicious sex a little fuzzy! Proceed with caution!

> **TIDBIT** Tequila, derived from the agave cactus, is the national drink of Mexico!

WATER

Ahhh… known universally as a life giver - water cleanses, refreshes, nourishes, sustains, and creates! Hot, cold, flavored, bottled, bubbly, or tap… drink it for the health and sustenance of your body and your baby!

WINE*

Wine is made from grapes… and both grapes and wine have been associated (in moderation, please!) with love, romance, lust, passion, and fertility throughout all ages. Wine relaxes our bodies while enhancing our senses, and there is even scientific evidence to suggest that red wine unclots veins… so see (and feel!) for yourself… where that blood rushes!

THE MORNING AFTER

Otherwise known as Breakfast!

CAFFEINE

See (or experience!) why coffee/tea are breakfast beverages of choice! Just one cup of coffee prior to love-making allegedly improves sperm motility! *Mister Coffee* takes on a whole new meaning!

♂ CINNAMON BUNS

Since cinnamon buns are known to increase penile blood flow by as much as 40%... you'll know the true meaning of "Good Morning!"

> **TIDBIT** Cinnamon has been mentioned in writings as far back as 2700 BC... no wonder!

♂ DOUGHNUTS

Want to keep his penile blood flow flowing? According to researchers at Chicago's Smell and Taste Treatment and Research Foundation, the scent of doughnuts causes the greatest increase in penile blood flow than of any food tested! Although a doughnut won't do much for his physique, it sure will rev him *up* again. Why not play your own version of horseshoes... toss him a doughnut (and if the doughnut *fits*, think about finding a new man)!

EGGS

Eggs... eggs... and more eggs! Whatever your preference in prepared eggs - eggs are, for obvious reasons, symbols of fertility... and eggs fall into the aphrodisiac category because of their magical nutritional values of protein, vitamins A and D, and iron. But perhaps most important for you, eggs stimulate sexual desire! So poach... scramble... fry... or boil - these "babies" are sure to get you over... easy!

> **TIDBIT** The yolk, eaten raw, is considered the most sexually potent part of the egg... but remember that there is increased risk of food-borne illness associated with raw eggs!

CHAPTER 7

Aromas

Nothing awakens the reminiscence like an odor!
- *VICTOR HUGO*

Aromas are everywhere. Aromas show up in many forms. And aromas, like food aphrodisiacs, are astonishingly easy to use every day! The same process of **stimuli ▶ testosterone ▶ nervous system ▶ pelvic region ▶ blood vessels ▶ erectile tissue** also applies to the sense of smell!

You already know the scents that drive you crazy (in a good way)! All you need do is apply the same aphrodisical principles to harness those olfactory delights! Is it his after-shave that *does it* for you? His shoe polish? His pillowcase? For your husband, is it your perfume? Your shampoo? Your favorite flower? Your apple (or pumpkin!) pie?

Whatever the stimulus, aromas all fall into the category of pheromones - virtually undetectable airborne "chemical" odors that transmit wonderful communications about such important things as... you guessed it... sex!

Remember... you're getting yourself ready for baby-making! It's supposed to be natural and fun and romantic and exciting! Now, we are not suggesting that the aromas from your favorite flowers, or your desired bath oils, or your preferred candles and incense will get you pregnant - but what we are saying is that the *stimulation* of these aromas, the magical reasons why you and your husband are drawn to certain scents (and to be scientific for a moment, your special *pheromones*), can enhance your love-making and your desire to do so.

We all know the expression *practice makes perfect*, but coming home from a stressful job, or a missed appointment, or in horrific traffic or inclement weather, only to arrive to a pile of laundry and a sink full of dishes... well, hop into bed under these circumstances, and even if your Basal Body Thermometer indicates "perfect"... all the *practicing* in the world isn't going to make anything *perfect*!

So to escape the day (or days) from hell...
May just mean capturing some tantalizing smells!

Accordingly to Allison England in her book ***Aromatherapy and Massage For Mother and Baby***, a woman's pheromones change with her menstrual cycle, becoming sweeter around ovulation. Her own sense of smell is more pronounced then too, no doubt to seek out a *musky* male. And apparently men also find women more attractive at this time... *ovulation*... as well. And it is also amazing to note that *puberty* brings on the male musk scent to which women are sexually drawn. But... you may find it fascinating, and even helpful to know that there are certain flowers, essential oils, candles, and incense that are reputed to spark up the sex drive as well!

Remember that all of this is relaxation *practice*, and delicious sex *practice*, is for that day or month or moment when you decide - *this is it*! It is time to try for a baby!

So arrange your flowers! Bathe in your oils! And light your fires! Allow aromas and scents to calm your ire!

THE FLOWER SHOP

The flower is the poetry of reproduction.

- *JEAN JIRANDOUX*

Flowers are not only a metaphor for the circle of life - from seed, to stalk, to bloom, and back again - but flowers also represent abundance, reproduction, fertility, and life.

The following flowers... let's call them *fertility flowers*... are as easy to procure as your favorite foods. Depending upon your region, simply snipping or picking or purchasing is all you need to do. And the ways in which you choose to use flowers are as limitless as your imagination - mix them, match them, fill rooms with them, spread petals on your bed or front hall or stairs - use flowers as they are intended... for romance and fertility!

DAFFODIL

Daffodils are feminine and ruled by the planet Venus. Rich in greens and yellows... they exude the symbols and colors of fertility and warm communication. As a touch of magic, Daffodils in the bedroom are reputed to increase fertility... for Daffodils, one of the first flowers of spring, represent rebirth. So, shall we say... *stalk* up!?

GERANIUM

Feminine, and ruled by Venus, Geraniums can be brought into your home in pots... or arranged, freshly cut, in vases. Place where, well... you feel like putting them, but the bedroom is especially lucky! And just so you know, *red* Geraniums strengthen health, *pink* Geraniums are often used in love spells... but as a touch of magic, use *white* Geraniums to increase fertility! You may even want to mix the colors... you know... for health, love, *and* fertility!

JASMINE

Beautiful and fragrant... often referenced by poets, Jasmine's sensual powers are reputed to boost a woman's sexual confidence up a notch! Cleopatra is said to have relied on the scent of Jasmine to announce to her lovers that she was approaching! Your new best friend around your home, and in your bedroom... may just have to be *Jasmine*!

> **TIDBIT** Flowers, arranged in *baskets*, are thought to symbolize and intensify both passion and fertility!

MISTLETOE

To shake things up a bit... and it usually takes a male presence to do so... bring on the Mistletoe! Mistletoe is masculine in gender, ruled by the sun, and traditionally known as the "kissing flower" at Christmas time. Legend tells us that kissing beneath a sprig of Mistletoe will keep your lover, but we can go even further than that... for as a touch of magic, women in ancient times carried Mistletoe to enhance conception. Hmmm... dare you hang Mistletoe in each room... during each season!?

PINE

Deliciously strong and masculine, and ruled by the planet Mars... the tall, strong Pine tree, with its giant testicle-shaped cones, is *very* sensual! And as a touch of magic, pinecones can be carried to increase fertility. Why? It's not just the vibrant masculine scent of Pine, but the symbolism in the shape of its fruit. Hmmm... is it the holiday season? Is there a Pine scent wafting around your home!? Fah-lah-lah-lah-lah-lah-lah-lah...! We hope you've been a very good girl this year!

> **TIDBIT** Pinecone-tipped wands were used as fertility symbols by the Greeks, and pinecone images have been found on excavated amulets.

ROSE

Really in a category of its own! Let's face it... what woman is going to turn away a dozen Roses delivered to her at work or at home? Or perhaps better yet, delivered by her husband in... well, nothing at all! Now why is this!? The Rose is the universal feminine love flower, associated with Venus, the planet of love. Fragrant and velvety - aromatic and tactile - the Rose has been in existence for literally millions of years. Legends have *grown* around the Rose! Myths have *grown* around the Rose! Philosophers and poets have *embraced* the Rose. And lovers? Cleopatra was said to have scattered Rose petals where Mark Antony walked (or... laid!), and the extracted oil of the Rose was once reserved for royalty only! Perhaps, though, the mysterious and romantic power of the Rose is really no mystery at all... for the Rose Hips in some Rose species contain upwards of 7,000 mg. of vitamin C per 100 grams of pulp! Considering that oranges contain about 50 mg. of vitamin C per 100 grams of pulp... that's a lotta' blood-pumping vitamin C! So arrange Rose bouquets... or spread Rose petals... or sip Rose Hip tea... to invoke sensual, delicious sex. Go on, ladies... inhale the delicious sweetness!

> **TIDBIT** The aroma of the rose is considered not only an anti-depressant, but a mood-enhancer as well.

SUNFLOWER

It shouldn't come as a surprise that the Sunflower is ruled by the sun... but it may surprise you to learn that Sunflowers are considered masculine in gender! And... because Sunflowers grow so tall, and continually look to the sun, they are reputed to increase fertility. Towering, strikingly beautiful and radiant, they are also said to grant wishes. So, as a touch of magic, women (and men) who wish to conceive should not only bring Sunflowers into their homes, but *eat* Sunflower seeds as well, for they are just brimming with fertility-potent phosphorus!

We have listed some flowers that are reputed to possess the powers to increase fertility... but if flowers are your *thing*, don't just stop with our suggested list. Embrace any flower that has the magical capacity to enhance the power of your relationship. Perhaps your wedding bouquet was comprised of Calla Lilies, Tulips, Daisies, Orchids, or Babies Breath. These scents alone may bring you back to a glorious, happy, romantic, sexy time in your relationship. Remember... go with whatever gets you in the mood for delicious, all-encompassing, multiple months of fun and romance, and (baby-making?!) sex!

Using the gifts and symbolism of flowers, *fertilize* your passions for each other!

ESSENTIAL OILS

We are astonished at thought, but sensation is equally wonderful.

- VOLTAIRE

So you're thinking of having a baby...

"Just relax and let it happen!" Perfect advice for any woman! But just how to relax... (better yet, the two of you together?)... in the most deliciously sexy ways?

Well... relax, indulge, pamper, and spoil...
By adding a drop (or two) of essential oil(s)!

Oils, used in ceremonial services and rituals for literally thousands of years, are simply "little" miracles. For your

TIDBIT The oils that we list can be purchased very easily online, in supermarkets, at specialty shops, and in department stores!

baby-planning (or baby-making) relaxation, we offer to you essential oils that, according to legend, spark the passion, offer the pleasure of tranquillity (yes... relaxation), and trigger much needed (and wanted) bodily responses! And as a touch of magic, the oils we mention are also known to enhance fertility (if that's what you desire!). The best part is that essential oils can be used in a variety of wonderful ways. Our favorite oils are used in baths and massages for sensual, stress-free sex! Baths and massages are two of the most deliciously sexy ways in which to relax... and, after all... that's what it's all about!

Romantic to the touch, as well as for the scent, try some of these enchanting oils. Be very romantic and sexy with them...

To aid in *conception* through relaxation, Allison England, in her book ***Aromatherapy and Massage For Mother and Baby***, recommends these fabulous massage oils:

- **Massage Oil for Her** - Add 15 drops of Geranium Oil, and 5 drops of Rose Oil, to 2½ tablespoons of Almond Oil. Mix well.
- **Massage Oil for Him** - Add 5 drops of Clary Sage Oil, 5 drops of Rose Oil, 5 drops of Geranium Oil, and 5 drops of either Sandalwood or Ylang-Ylang Oil, to 2½ tablespoons of Almond Oil. Mix well.

Pay special attention to the lower back, abdomen, groin, and hip areas.

A WORD TO THE WISE:

We emphasize - a *strong* word to the wise... do not apply oil mixtures directly to your genital areas, as they may burn! Ouchy!

GERANIUM OIL

Geranium Oil is an aromatic oil with many properties. Its toning action works on the entire body - both male and female - and it also balances hormonal action on the *reproductive system* (lovely!). The scent is so attractive and popular... don't stop at oil - go for lotions, creams, soaps, sprays, etc... ! Geramium is the perfect scent oil for any time that you wish to dispel anxiety, or when stress may be a factor. Allow this bath or massage oil, or scent, to relax every part of your being... and then... give in to your desires!

JASMINE OIL

Considered both uplifting and simultaneously calming, Jasmine is not only an aphrodisical scent, but it is reputed to help in *preconception* and baby-making care... particularly because it gets your blood pumping to all of your important parts!

> **TIDBIT** Apparently Cleopatra knew the magic of Jasmine... as she seduced Antony by bathing in its oils.

MUSK OIL

Known as the love oil!... repeat, love oil!... Musk Oil scent is used not only to increase sensual passion, but to also invigorate sexual pleasure! Why not see if Musk lives *up* to its name!?

PATCHOULI OIL

Described as an "earthy" aroma, Patchouli Oil is considered a high-sexual-energy aphrodisiac that lifts your spirits while it diminishes anxiety. Its reputed properties - growth, *fertility*, success - are all excellent for baby-making!

A WORD TO THE WISE:

Use Patchouli Oil in moderation... as doses too large lead to sleepy-time!

ROSE OIL

The scent of Rose Oil, hugely aphrodisical in quality (that's right… it gets the blood flowing!), works miracles in both men and women. Seemingly always associated with either Venus or Aphrodite, the scent of Rose not only gets you begging for more, but it is reputed (ah ha!) to cure PMS in women and impotency in men! Your greatest dilemma - do you use your Rose Oil *before… during…* or *after…* your Rose Oil massage!? And as a touch of magic, try *Lady Luck Oil - 4 drops Sandalwood Oil, 7 drops Rose Oil, 5 drops Lavender Oil. Romany women were said to anoint their clothing with Lady Luck Oil to ensure success when hawking or fortune-telling. It is also used on candles and money.* **The Good Spell Book**, *Gillian Kemp*

> **TIDBIT** Beyond bath and massage… try leaving your favorite sexy scents on your linens or clothing, inside your husband's briefcase, on his computer keys, and even in his car! Just be careful that the enchantment doesn't distract him too much! We mean, he (and you!) might need to actually *work* once-in-awhile!

SANDALWOOD OIL

Sandalwood Oil has a wonderful, relaxing, aphrodisical aroma, and it is known for its affectiveness on male impotency! Use this oil for the ultimate sense of relaxation… the release of your daily stresses… the awakening of his senses! *Wood* you dare!?

VANILLA OIL

If lusty energy is what you're looking for, bring on the Vanilla Oil! Sensual, smooth, seductive, and soothing… like a vanilla ice cream cone on a hot summer night… except you'll be *glad* you're not a kid anymore! Va-voom!

YLANG-YLANG OIL

Exotic, mysterious, romantic… Ylang-Ylang Oil is not only an aphrodisiac, but it is used to calm and relax your nervous system. It increases male potency, and "it" (the scent and/or the experience!) stays with you all day long! And as a touch of magic, try *Lucky Planet Oil by combining 5 drops Ylang-Ylang Oil, 3 drops Clary Sage Oil, and 5 drops Geranium Oil. Lucky Planet Oil rubbed on an orange candle, which is then left to burn down, is said to encourage a lucky turn of events.* **The Good Spell Book**, *Gillian Kemp*

The aromas of Essential Oils cause powerful psychological and physiological responses in our bodies. With the oils we've mentioned, there is virtually no work for you to do. As you breathe in the aromas, your nose sends messages to the brain, which in turn send quick and strong impulses that affect your hormones, sensual feelings, and heart rates. This is why you will feel so relaxed… and calm enough to concentrate on what needs to be done! The *relaxation* part is the key! The oils are *essential* because they help in preventing "things" from cluttering your mind or affecting your senses!

Let the rest of the world disappear as you bathe together, massage one another, and allow your love and your passions to take over.

Enjoy these nights as often as you can in your preparation to create a baby…!

CANDLES AND INCENSE

What can give us surer knowledge than our senses?

- Lucretius

Sensual intimacy between a husband and wife knows no *bounds*… and sexual desire may not know *time*… but the actual time/work restraints on two separate lives generally make the night time the passionate time. To offset the darkness of night, we have been blessed with candles. And to bring the earth's vibrations into our homes, we have been blessed with incense…

many of which, if you choose to believe, possess fertility magic! So throw "common scents" to the wind, ladies (and guys), and read on!

Whether from Mother Earth or Heaven sent…
Get turned on to colors and scents!

CANDLES*

And we're not talking about your husband forgetting to pay the electric bill, or the Blackout of 2003! We're talking romance - you know, candles along the mantel… candles blazing a path to your bedroom door… candles on your night stand… candles around your bathtub… all in preparation to get you and your husband in the mood for looovvvveee. So… to enhance your practice for baby-making… why not first know the *secrets* of candle *color!?*

**Always remember to extinguish your candles prior to leaving your home or retiring for the evening… and as a touch of magic, always extinguish your candles with a snuffer, or with your moistened fingers, so as not to "blow" your wishes away!*

COLORS!

RED immediately arouses passionate and emotional energy. To the Romans, red was the color of masculine arousal (hmmm…), so use it as the color that rushes his blood to his face… sends his blood coursing through his body… and races his blood, to… well… you know where! So do yourself (and believe us, *him* too!)

a favor and start using red candles! And for further arousal, incorporate the color red into your home! Add red pillows to your bedroom… red towels to the bathroom… red placemats to the dinner table… red "throws" to the living room…! Just the sight of the color red may get you in the mood! Hey… it's worth a try!

GREEN is the color of nature… of creativity… of growth and reproduction… and hence, is known as the color of fertility. Now, you could have delicious sex on the green of some golf course, on your husband's high school football field, or in the stadium seats of Fenway Park's Green Monster (yes, we're Red Sox fans!)… but even though you may be fulfilling your man's greatest fantasy, you'd both probably be arrested… so just save yourself the hassle and buy some green candles! And just as we suggested with the color *red*, add some splashes of *green* to your home… anywhere that inspires you to do so!

RED AND GREEN COLOR SCENTS

Use your ***"Scents" and Sensibility!*** Further enhance the lusty candle color variations of **reds** and **greens** with *scents* of passion and fertility. Add the following delicious scents to your home whenever you can… so they too can work their magic!

APPLE

An Apple a day does more than keep the doctor away! Embraced by many cultures, the apple is celebrated as anything from a *love charm* to a magical object… from a *symbol of fruitfulness* to a token of knowledge. Let the Apple scent waft through your Home Sweet Home!

BALSAM FIR

Ever green - hence, the term "Evergreen" - the Fir tree is considered the tree of birth in Irish folklore... and in Finland, the Balsam Fir is sacred to the family. Rich in both color and scent, you may not want to bring this scent into the bedroom until you're *absolutely* ready to conceive!

CINNAMON

Cinnamon is one of those "sugar and spice and everything nice" scents! Highly prized and valued in Eastern and Western trade, and mentioned in literature from earliest times, the scent of Cinnamon increases sensual desire. Come on, ladies... sprinkle liberally!

SAGE

Sage is not only a soothing shade of green, but it is referenced in writings from both ancient Greece and Rome! Sage scent has forever been used to strengthen the vitality of the brain, and, well... *muscles* (which can only be helpful for your purposes!).

STRAWBERRY

Known as a plant of Venus, the Goddess of Love, Strawberries invoke both luck and love. Just how lucky will you get with this scent!?

Although we list several, don't restrict yourself to just these scents! As we say... throw common "scents" to the wind, and utilize your favorite illuminates - no matter what color, size, or scent! You know your favorite scents... and you probably know your husband's favorite scents - perhaps pumpkin pie?... lavender?... coffee?... watermelon?... mint?... lemon?... maybe even butterscotch?... to name but a few!

Scents encompass time and seasons and emotions and memories special to each of you, as well as the two of you together! We listed some lusty, fertility reds and greens, but your passions and powers and personal preferences are as individual as your marriage.

So experiment! Enjoy! **Relax!**

INCENSE

The word incense means *to inflame, to excite, to kindle a passion or ardent feeling* - to... shall we say, bring us into our senses! For your purposes, incense in the forms of cones, sticks, or pulverized herbs may be exactly what you need or desire in order to inflame, excite, and kindle your passion!

> **TIDBIT** Incense sticks and candles, when burned, combine the powerful elements of *Fire* energy and *Earth* energy... which are known to influence creativity and emotions. Ahhh!... perfect for baby-making!

Incense products can easily be purchased online, from specialty stores, or even in many supermarkets, but some people enjoy the magical powers of mixing their own plant materials to create special incense blends. Be our guests... just as long as you know what you are doing! But to make things easy for those of you who just wish to enjoy the scents and symbolism of incense - for some recognizable suggestions, read on...

FOR THAT LOVEY-DOVEY FEELING, TRY...

Amber	Rosemary
Gardenia	Strawberry
Jasmine	Violet
Lavender	Ylang Ylang

FOR THAT LUSTY FEELING, TRY...

Cinnamon	Peppermint
Clove	Saffron
Ginger	Vanilla
Patchouli	

AND IF IT'S TIME TO VENTURE INTO FERTILITY, TRY...

Basil	Rose
Mistletoe	Sandalwood
Musk Root	

There are hundreds of varieties of incense... and hundreds more incense blends. All incense varieties contain *properties*, whether you believe them to be magical or not... and many of these properties are interchangeable. For example, Rose Incense can be burned for love, lust, or fertility. Again, this preconception journey is fun, exciting, sexy, and meaningful... a time of new beginnings, of growth, and awareness. So enjoy a new scent or two, and even if your husband is experiencing incense for the first time - live it up, down, and sideways... just relax and enjoy the deliciously sexy-scented atmosphere!

CHAPTER 8

Herb Magic

Sex, pleasure and women... Is a kind of magic spell.
– *SIMONE DE BEAUVOIR*

Ahhh... herbs! Not just for cooking in the kitchen! What you'll be reading here is pretty much lore that has been passed from generation to generation by oral and written traditions. Sometimes the medical world scoffs at the teachings of herbal medicines and cures and remedies, but... you know what?...there is just something to be said for different approaches used throughout the world, among multiple cultures of people, for virtually thousands of years.

Herbal powers are historically fascinating, extremely interesting, perhaps exotic, and maybe even *necessary* to add to your life! All of the herbs that we mention can be purchased online, in specialty and department stores... and most can be purchased right in your supermarket - or better yet, nurtured on a sunny windowsill or in your own herb garden!

We're touching only upon herbs known for their powers and properties of love, lust, and fertility... so you just may want to hang a little sign on your door...

Do not disturb...
Using powerful lust and fertility herbs!

And we simply must start with Ginseng and Mandrake, both *human-shaped* roots... and considered powerful because of that particular human-shaped phenomenon!

GINSENG

The Chinese word Ginseng actually means *image of man*. Ginseng has been used for thousands of years to increase virility in men, and to increase sexual appetite! Ginseng tea is still used today to induce lust! Tea for two, anyone!? Ginseng is also reputed to possess the power to grant wishes, so as a touch of magic, carry the Ginseng Root to attract love or lust; or visualize your wish on a Ginseng Root and then toss it (the Ginseng Root, not your lover) into running water!

MANDRAKE

A WORD TO THE WISE:

Stay away from the Mandrake Root unless it is in the *form* of an amulet carved to *resemble* a Mandrake Root! Mandrake Root has been used for centuries in magic potions, but it is now known to be *poisonous*. Yes, *poisonous*.

Because of its human shape, Mandrake Root is believed to contain powerful and curative powers of fertility, love, and protection. And also because of its human shape, Mandrake has been used as a symbol of fertility in many cultures. As a touch of magic, a Mandrake Root (and again, *carved*... not real!) may be placed on your mantel or headboard to deliver its fertility and love magic.

And now to the others...

BODHI

All right... have you ever seen a Bodhi Tree? Or perhaps you have and just don't know it... but it is sacred to Vishnu, one of the principal Hindu deities, who is identified as the preserver of the world. Maybe this is why the Bodhi Tree is so highly regarded in the East as a symbol of fertility! And legend has it that if a barren woman walks naked (ooh-la-la!) beneath a Bodhi Tree, she will magically become fertile. Could be worth a try! Just be discreet... so as not to alarm your neighbors!

CHICKWEED

First, let us just say... Chickweed is known for its *upright*, round stalks. Yummy! But don't eat it... rather *carry* Chickweed for its magical powers of lust, love, fertility, and potency!

CORIANDER (Chinese Parsley, Cilantro)

In case you discover that you are pregnant while reading this book, you may want to start seasoning with Coriander, for its magical properties are reputed to make your future children ingenious! Our philosophy... just start using it now! Why wait!?

CUCKOO FLOWER

OK... this is a real fun one! The name Cuckoo Flower is given to several wild flowers that are in bloom in Spring... flowers such as Blue Bells, Ragged Robins, Buttercups, Marsh Marigolds, Cow Slips, Lady's Smocks, Wood Sorrel, and Wild Hyacinth. Now, this is the fertility part... a Cuckoo Bird is known by the call of the male during mating time (the word *cuckoo* is the imitation of the sound)! Perhaps "cuckoo - cuckoo" may become your secret mating code!? As a touch of magic, the *tubers* of these flowers can be carried or worn to promote conception - large *tubers* when wishing for a boy, smaller *tubers* for a girl!

> **TIDBIT** A *tuber* is an underground structure consisting of a solid, thickened out-growth of the stem... think of a potato with its little (or big!) lumps and roots.

DOCK

When a woman ties Dock seeds to her left arm, it is said that she will conceive a child. Arts and craft project, anyone!?

GRAINS OF PARADISE

We'll get right into the magic! Known as a powerful wishing herb, you may want to follow this Grains of Paradise ritual in a wish for a healthy baby:

> *Hold the Grains of Paradise in your hands and make a wish... then take small pieces of the herb and toss them in each direction - beginning in the North, tossing and turning clockwise - and ending in the West. Wish hard and truly believe as you perform this magic ritual!*

HAZEL (Nuts)

We love anything that has to do with nuts! According to Celtic legend... the bushy shrub known as the Tree of Knowledge yields edible Hazel nuts that increase fertility when *carried*!

HORSETAIL

Giddy-up! Ride em' cowgirl! You may even want to get yourself stirrups and a cowgirl hat for this herb! Consisting of slender branches and jointed stems... this plant resembles, as one may guess, a *horsetail*! Placed in the bedroom, Horsetail increases fertility. We wonder why!? There is also the female Horsetail, called the *Mares-tail*, which is a smaller version of Horsetail. So don't feel left out, boys... grab your cowboy gear and *ride* until she calls, "Whoa boy!"

LAVENDER

The way to use this sweet-scented romantic herb is to simply wear it as a perfume, and/or (if you're particularly literary... listen up, guys!) write a love note and rub the paper with Lavender. This has been known to attract your lover in the most lustful of ways... so no wonder Lavender has been referred to as a "precious herb" as early as the 16th century! Start *spraying* and *writing* and *rubbing*... !

OAK

Hmmm... something strong, long, and solid... we like it already! The most worshiped tree on earth, the Oak symbolizes great strength and triumph over adversity. Some Indian cultures revered the acorn, the fruit of the Oak, as a symbol of fertility... and it is said, that as a touch of magic, carrying an acorn increases fertility and sexual potency. As a matter of fact, in some European countries, Oak boughs were often carried at wedding ceremonies as symbols of great fertility. Sounds *oak-ay* to us!

DATE PALM TREE

Our favorite as a warm climate tree! Considered the Tree of Life by the Egyptians, Chinese, and Hindus, the Date Palm Tree is a marvelous giver of fruit. In fact, such an abundance of fruit is produced that the Date Palm Tree is considered a fertility tree... especially considering its unusually upright stem (OK... yummy)! If you are near one... well, do whatever you wish beneath it... we'll never tell! Or, just *eat* the date(s) to enhance fertility! As a touch of magic, have your husband carry a date nut, or just stick one in his pocket... to increase sexual potency!

PATCHOULI

The word itself meaning "green leaf"... Patchouli is a versatile plant that yields an essential oil scent used for perfumes. And as a touch of magic, the leaves can be carried as a fertility talisman. Because of its lust-inducing aromatic scent, Patchouli is frequently used in baths and sachets for such savory purposes! You will truly love Patchouli's magic!

POMEGRANATE (Yes, we know it's a fruit!)

As magical as any herb, the Pomegranate is a highly regarded and miraculous fertility symbol because of its abundance of seeds. In many cultures, women have eaten the seeds of the Pomegranate while wishing for children... and the rind of the Pomegranate is carried for the same wish. The Pomegranate is also a symbol of hope, for if you wish ardently before eating one, your wish may be granted! As a touch of magic, if a woman breaks a Pomegranate into a circle drawn on the ground, the number of seeds that scatter outside the circle indicates the number of children she will have... interesting! Just make sure you perform this "juicy" touch of magic outdoors! Also, because of the Pomegranate's association with romance, love, and children - poets have mused about it for centuries. As early as 1541, one poet wrote, "Ye must give him some of a Pomegranate to eat." Good advice!

POPPY SEEDS

Use your best judgment with poppy. Yes, it is a fertility enhancer... but alas, it is also known as a sleep inducer. Do you want a *sizzling* night, or a night of ZZZZZZs!? Perhaps you may wish to use Poppy Seeds to stimulate fertility, and then consume some again to *rest up* for your next passionate encounter!

SESAME

Shall we say, "Open Sesame!?" After all, *you* are the treasure!

This magical herb contains seeds which can be used as food, or yielded into cooking and/or anointing oils. But you might want to mix your Sesame Seeds with a touch of honey to create Phallic Cakes… yes, we said Phallic Cakes!… that resemble the female reproductive organ - HELLO! - as was done in ancient times to promote fertility! Perhaps you should teach your husband the magic pass phrase - "Open Sesame" - to obtain admission!

SOUTHERNWOOD

First… we just enjoy this name! Second, this hardy plant is known throughout Europe, North America, and Asia, but is sometimes called Lad's Love or Boy's Love. But beyond that… whether *your* "Boy's Wood" is northern, southern, eastern, or western, this plant is known to arouse lustful feelings when placed under your bed! So… get that *wood working*!

WHEAT

Cultivated since the beginning of time… and reproduced year after year and generation after generation… Wheat is known universally as a symbol of fruitfulness and fertility. Multiple rituals have arisen around the planting, sowing, and harvesting of Wheat Germ. So it makes sense, that as a touch of magic, Wheat *carried* or *eaten* has become known as a potent fertility enhancer.

MORE HERBAL POWER

And believe it or not, we (perhaps) have saved the best Herbal Powers for last!

OK… so you may have baked Phallic Cakes… be seasoning with Chinese Parsley and Cilantro… laying in beds of Cuckoo Flowers or Horsetail! You may have massaged Lavender on each others' bodies… and possibly even whet your sensual appetites with Hazelnuts and Poppy Seeds…

But there's more!

According to Susun S. Weed, author of ***Wise Woman Herbal for the Childbearing Year*** (now in its 29th Printing!), herbs used to encourage a pregnancy are characterized by their ability to: 1) nourish and tonify the uterus; 2) nourish the entire body; 3) relax the nervous system; 4) establish and balance normal functioning of the hormonal system; and 5) balance sexual desire.

Herbal wisdom lies in its natural simplicity! Who could ask for more!? Discover, or *rediscover* the wisdom of Susan Weed's words and advice in these recommended herbs:

RED CLOVER FLOWERS

This is the single most useful herb for establishing fertility. Its high vitamin content is especially useful for the uterus; its high protein content aids the entire body; its profuse and exceedingly absorbable calcium and magnesium relax the nervous system and promote fertility; its high mineral content, including virtually every trace mineral needed by the glands, helps restore and balance hormonal functions. In addition, Red Clover alkalinizes the body and may balance the acid/alkaline level of the vagina and uterus in favor of conception.

Red Clover is often combined with Peppermint in fertility brews since Mints are safe and pleasant tasting sexual stimulants.

Infuse one ounce of Red Clover blossoms and a teaspoon of Peppermint (or any other Mint) in a quart of water for four hours. This infusion may be taken freely throughout the day and for several months continuously.

NETTLE

Nettle is a uterine tonic and general nourisher with a special ability to strengthen the kidneys and adrenals. Its high mineral and chlorophyll content makes it an excellent food and tonic for the hormonal system. These characteristics make Nettle infusions a wonderful brew for increasing fertility.

As with Red Clover, drink one or more cups of the infusion daily for several months.

RED RASPBERRY LEAVES

Raspberry leaves are another wonderful choice as an herbal fertility promoter. It is most effective when combined with Red Clover.

One or more cups of the infusion (prepared by steeping one half ounce of Red Clover blossoms and one half ounce of Raspberry leaves in a quart of water for four hours) can be taken daily and continued for months. Another way to increase the fertility promoting ability of Raspberry is to add 15-20 drops of either Dong Quai root tincture or False Unicorn root tincture to each cup of Raspberry leaf infusion.

DONG QUAI ROOT

This is widely and highly regarded as a fertility promoter. The form that is favored is a water-based combination extract sold under the name "Tang Kwei Gin". Best results are obtained when Dong Quai preparations are taken during the days between ovulation and menstruation, and discontinued from the beginning of the menstrual flow to ovulation.

~

For some of you, the use of herbs may be brand new. For others of you, Herbal Powers and Herbal Magic may already be a part of your lives. Whichever it may be… remember that herbs bring wisdom, health, power, and fertility to the lives of those who believe!

CHAPTER 9

Amulets

We cannot afford to miss any advantage.

- RALPH WALDO EMERSON

Would you ever have thought that buying your husband a little toy bull might charge up every sexual molecule in his body!? Well… this is no bull! The reason is not only fun, but also interesting, historically based, and incredibly, deliciously sexy…!

Your little bull (or big bull, depending upon *your* man!) is, or could be, considered an amulet. Amulets are material objects created to represent the characteristics of the desired object. From primitive times to the present day, people have worn or carried amulets, or placed amulets in their homes, in order to bring certain powers or wishes. The object, or the amulet, creates a positive energy focus, positive thoughts, and complete physical and emotional awareness and concentration in making your wish come true.

For your purposes… we're calling on all fertility *animals*,

So depending upon your choice of pet(s)…
Use one, *or all*, as amulets!

BULL

OK... back to the bull! When you think *bull*, you probably think masculine, strong, fierce, competitive, powerful, fast, and sexual prowess. Well, you're not alone! The Persians, Greeks, Romans, Hittites, and Zulus also saw the bull in the same way... and used the bull in great stories and myths of strength, maleness, and reproductive powers (obviously our favorite!). So it should come as no surprise that wearing a bull amulet, or (surprise! surprise!) placing a bull under your bed, is considered a fertility enhancer. This should be particularly enticing for you Tauruses out there!

FISH

Although fish and shells are traditionally not considered *animals*, keep in mind that to concentrate on your wish of having a baby... you may just need some fish or shells! When it comes down to it (it's pretty simple, ladies), the shape of the fish is phallic, or masculine... and the shape of the shell is feminine. Many cultures associate fish with fertility because of the abundance of these creatures... but also because fish contain such fertility inducing vitamins and minerals (but we're not talking about *eating* them in this chapter!). The salmon, in particular, is associated with fertility because of its incredible determination in finding its spawning grounds. And the scallop (female), well... first of all, it resembles the vulva (yes, we said vulva)... and it also symbolizes marriage, passion, and fertility. Be creative with your fish and shell amulets! Wear them on necklaces, bracelets, or earrings. Decorate with them... think wallpaper, pot holders, towels, paintings and prints, glass sculptures... we could go on and on! Enjoy their tranquillity, their peace, their magic. Who knows?... perhaps even a bedroom aquarium?

FROG

Do you remember the wonderful story of the "Frog Prince"...

where the frog, having been kissed by a princess, turns back into a prince!? Well, we can't document this occurrence in *real* life... but all over the world folktales have combined stories of these frog/prince transformations that associate the frog, simply by being kissed, with princely love, marriage, and happiness. Perhaps the frog is considered so magical because it lays numerous eggs at one time?... or that its great *fecundity* (meaning fertile, fruitful and productive) inspires the *confidence* of fertility and abundance? Whatever the reason, bring a frog into your "kingdom" as a fertility enhancer, and he may just turn your husband into your own "Frog Prince" for the night! Hey, maybe a possible mating call could be... "Ribbit!"!

GOAT

It may surprise you to learn that this little barnyard creature is considered a fertility symbol. It sure surprised us! We mean, have you ever seen a goat up-close and personal!? We have... and enough said. But, in any case... goats have been considered fertility-bringers in many cultures, and therefore considered viable wedding gifts... (what a lucky bride!). Actually, Aphrodite herself made the goat a sacred animal, for it was her transportation of choice! So... be our guest to wear or carry a goat amulet, or place a goat amulet somewhere in your home. Heck, if you have a live goat, you're already ahead of the game! And for you Capricornians, this is a very favorable amulet.

RABBIT

So maybe those famous, sexy, bunny ears and cottontails weren't too many steps removed from the magic of passion and fertility!? Both prolific and plentiful, rabbits and hares have been associated with love, fertility, the menstrual cycle, the circle of life, and even the moon for hundreds of years. In fact, it was thought at one time in China that female rabbits became pregnant by simply staring at the moon! And reiterating its proliferation qualities, the female rabbit is capable of delivering up to six litters a year!... and she takes very special care in preparing and protecting her nest, and also seems to truly enjoy her colonies of large families. Think about it... just as you are preparing your "nest" for a natural, yet miraculous event, so too are rabbits everywhere. Why not bring a rabbit amulet into your nest... for this powerful force of motherhood just may get you *hopping*! And as a touch of magic, since the first day of any month offers a fresh start, one lucky New England custom is to say the word "rabbits" as the very first word of the month! A variation of this custom is to say the words "white rabbits" three times as the *last* words you say on the eve of the new month... and say the word "hares" three times upon awakening on the first day of the new month! All three charms are said to ensure a month that is filled with magic and good luck!

UNICORN

Although a mythical beast... perhaps the luckiest of all amulets is the unicorn! Come on, ladies... the long, slender horn alone is allegedly up to 36 inches - let's see... in our calculations, that's about 6 men - preferably 5 on a good day! But seriously speaking... if we can be serious about a unicorn... it is commonly associated with love, and said to be tamed by the touch of a virgin. The unicorn is also a desired fertility symbol because the unicorn is both powerful, yet gentle, at the same time - qualities that most of us adore. To stimulate fertility and arouse sexual desire, unicorn amulets should be worn as jewelry. And for fun... we guess... you could *pretend* you're a virgin... about to make love with your lover for the very first time! It's up to you just how far you want to take the unicorn magic!

STORK

Ah!... could a discussion of fertility not include, arguably, the most widely recognized symbol of delivered bundles of joy - the stork!? Known for its raucous, beak-striking mating performances, the stork represents great hope, great luck, and rebirth!

OLD WIVES' TALE: If a stork builds a nest in your chimney, you will have a boy!

CHAPTER 10

Sex & Fertility Symbols

A person gets from a symbol the meaning he puts into it.
- *JUSTICE ROBERT JACKSON*

Nuts? Giant penises? Interlocking triangles? Breast lifting? Well... in a word, *yes*! *Thumbs up* to all of these and many more!

Both historically and culturally, symbols identify a particular object, image, or gesture with an established meaning... and sex and fertility are no exceptions! Actually... quite the contrary... there are so many sex and fertility symbols that it's difficult for us to even narrow down the list! So, without further adieu, here are some of our favorites... and better yet, some of these can easily be used as fertility *amulets* as well...

So to have your Baby wishes fulfilled...
Look to meaningful fertility symbols!

PHALLIC GIANT

We'll start with our favorite - the Phallic Giant! We've mentioned this sexy symbol throughout the book… but now you'll be formally introduced to him! And yes, as we're sure you've imagined, it is a *him*! A *very big* him! The actual word *phallus* is the Greek word for *penis*, and it means "an image of the male generative organ, symbolizing the generative power in nature." We'll put it to you this way… you may not want to walk around with one of these hanging around your neck, for they are images of giants with giant erect penises! But in many cultures, Phallic Giants represent fertility and the masculine power of creation… which would account for the erect penis, we're sure! Phallic Giants were often carved in stone and/or wood, and used for the exact symbol for which they represented - fertility and sex. We hope you're lucky enough to not need a carved symbol… for you have your very own, in-the-flesh, Phallic Giant at home!

> **TIDBIT** Priapus, the son of Aphrodite, is considered a God of fertility and is best known for his - dare we say - 12-inch, perpetually erect penis! Everywhere Priapus went, plants and animals reproduced. Hmm… sounds pretty *cocky*, huh!?

EGG

Beyond hard-boiled, scrambled, or poached… eggs, since the beginning of time, have been celebrated all over the world as life-giving fertility symbols. On a romantic and spiritual level, the egg stands for *potential* life and the *continuity* of life. But for your purposes, let's be realistic - eggs are shaped like, hmmm… think of your husband standing in the nude. What jumps to mind!? - **testicles!** And as a touch of magic, a bride entering her new home should *break an egg* to ensure fertility!

ACORN (also see page 131 - *Oak*)

As some say, "Good things come in small packages!" - well,

consider the acorn one such package! As the fruit of the Oak tree, the acorn has long been considered a symbol of fertility. The Oak tree is prolific in producing its nuts (pun intended), but the acorn itself is also revered for the time it takes (up to three years) for one acorn to mature, expressing the idea that it takes *effort* to *achieve*. The acorn is also associated with Armetis, the Greek Goddess of fertility, marriage, and childbirth, and the protector of women and children ... and to whom these fruits of nature were dedicated. As a touch of magic, *carry* the potent little acorn... place them in baskets... or *wear* an acorn amulet to inspire thoughts of motherhood. Nothing could be more romantically simple!

> **TIDBIT** According to Canadian researcher Anthony Perks and published in the February 2003 issue of Britain's ***Journal of the Royal Society of Medicine***... the Stonehenge mystery has been solved! Perks writes that the configuration of stones represent the labia minora, the labia majora, the clitoris and the birth canal - a mother of the Earth Goddess who symbolically offered both "life and livelihood". (Perks, A. M., Bailey, D. M.: Stonehenge: a view from medicine. JRSocMed 2003; 96:94 - 98). Looks like some true fertility experts lived somewhere between 3000 and 1600 BC!

CORN DOLL

OK ladies, you may never think of corn-on-the-cob the same way again! Since sheaves of corn or sheaves of wheat are known fertility symbols because of their association with the earth, the sun, the sustenance of mankind, and celebrations of "breaking bread" (never mind the actual shape of an ear of corn!), it makes perfect sense that corn would find its way into a fertility symbol... the *corn doll*. And just how does one go about acquiring a corn doll!? Well, take an ear of corn... put a dress on it (yes, we actually said to dress it up!)... make the head, arms, and legs from the corn stalks - and voila! Your corn doll... or ones like it... have been used for hundreds of years as fertility symbols by women wishing to conceive. Hang yours in your home… for it's not as *corny* as it may sound!

CORNUCOPIA

And speaking of corn, let's talk about the cornucopia… because, after all, you probably never thought of the sexual nature and symbolism of this long, hard, thick, eye-catching, yet hollow (OK… so we're getting a little carried away!) Thanksgiving decoration that you place on the table across from your mother-in-law every year! But in fact, the cornucopia, sometimes called the *horn of plenty* (hmm… we won't even touch that!) is the perfect symbol of male and female, as it is both phallic as well as hollow. And still more! When filled with fruits, the cornucopia further symbolizes greater fertility, and is reputed to grant wishes to its possessor. As a touch of magic, fill a cornucopia with fertility fruits (see pages 99 - 103). It is the *perfect* fertility symbol! So be bold! Don't just fill one in the fall - use cornucopias in seasons all! What will your mother-in-law say!?

MAY POLE

And speaking of seasons, let's jump to spring! You may not be able to erect (pun intended!) a May Pole in your own backyard… OK, maybe you will!… but you may find it interesting to know that the May Pole, a phallic symbol in itself, became part of spring fertility rituals in many European and North American cultures because of its perfect shape! Great care was taken to decorate the May Pole… and celebrations and dances and feasts became part of the fertility ritual. But don't fret if it's not spring, and you don't own a *real* May Pole… we're sure you can design your own celebrations around your own *May Pole* every night!

> TIDBIT
> **May Day**
> May 1st, sometimes referred to as *Beltane*, began in Europe as a celebration of sexual enticement!

SHAPES

From the simplest to the most elaborate, shapes occurring as symbols appear within every culture and religion known to man! These shapes contain such powerful spiritual, psychological, and emotional associations that they have been known to create a dramatic impact on the hopes and prayers and lives of those who believe. Keep your eyes open for these often commonly recognized, yet wonderful fertility symbols... or *wear* these "shapes" as fertility amulets:

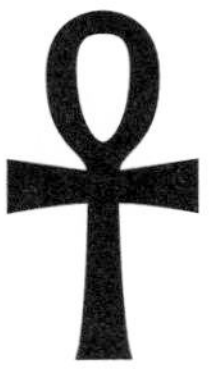

Ankh - An Egyptian symbol, the ankh is comprised of a cross with a looped top (representing both male and female), and was known as a symbol of the regeneration of life... hence, it is still known as the *key of life*. The ankh symbol is said to enhance both physical and spiritual fertility, and has the power to unlock the mysteries of heaven and earth.

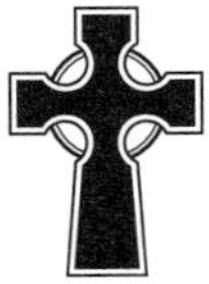

Celtic Cross - This shape combines the cross with the circle... a true symbolic association of fertility, for the cross represents the male reproductive power and the circle represents the female reproductive power.

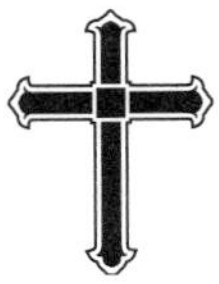

The Cross - The vertical line of the Cross represents the masculine, or heavenly principle... and the intersecting horizontal line represents the Earth, or feminine principle. The actual point of intersection is the symbolic meeting of heaven and earth... and mankind itself is the result of this union.

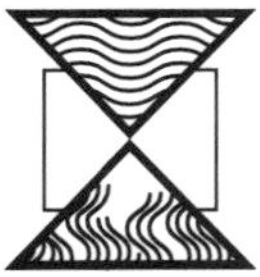

PointePointe - 2 triangles, 1 upward and 1 downward, placed point to point. The *upward* triangle symbolizes the male (of course!) in its association with fire, and the downward triangle is associated with the female, symbolizing water; *combined*, perfect balance and unity!

The Shape of the Letter M - As with any interlocking union, the M is formed by two interlocking points, indicative of the union of male and female.

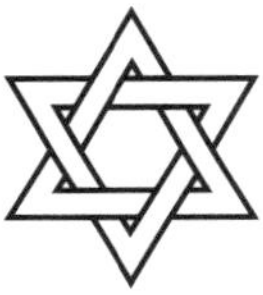

Seal of Solomon - The interlocking of the upward male triangle and the downward female triangle - each triangle interlocks with the other in perfect harmony… as do you and your husband.

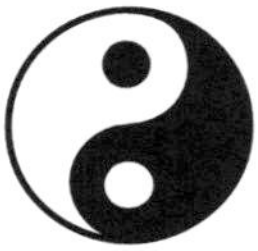

Tai Chi or Yin Yang - This Eastern symbol associates complete balance, carrying both the male (right) and the female (left)… as each side is a necessary force in the production of all forms, including children.

Now, there are virtually thousands of shapes that represent various religions, cultures, myths, legends, and folktales… we've named but a few. For a fascinating study of your own religious or cultural roots, and to provide stories to pass on to your own children… why not investigate your own significant or sacred shapes in your lives, including Coats of Arms, Runes, religious symbols, or perhaps even the shapes of the letters in your names!

GESTURES

Lifting of the Breasts

And no... this is not a typo! This symbol, as a *fertility gesture*, should probably remain reserved for the bedroom! But... to convey fertility as did Goddess Ishtar (the Babylonian Goddess of Lust and Sex who ruled over the Earth's fertility... and a woman no less!), you need only your hands and breasts! Lift and shake them, baby!... preferably with your husband as your audience!

Thumbs Up

And last but not least, *Thumbs Up* for the guys! Although the "thumbs up" gesture of today generally indicates *agreement* or *cheers* or *well done*... the "thumbs up" sign originated as a symbol of masculine virility! Come on... the shape of the thumb facing up... it's a no-brainer! What else can we say, guys... but *Thumbs Up*!

CHAPTER 11

Gems & Stones

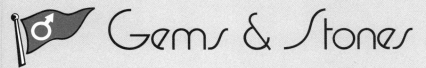

It is a great piece of skill to know how to guide your luck even while waiting for it.
- *Baltasar Gracian*

Diamonds may be a girl's best friend… but how do they compete with other gems and stones for lust and fertility!? The use of gems and stones for their magical properties has been in practice for thousands of years… and although we're not saying that your husband must run to the nearest jeweler, the Red Flag is for… oh, let's see… if he's feeling inspired for birthdays, anniversaries, holidays… or just some amazing fertility surprise!

For in the case that he buys a stone or a gem…
He should at least be aware of the powers in them!

As with all gems and stones, prices vary according to stone… size… clarity… etc., but keep in mind that most gems and stones can be represented by even the tiniest of specimens! Size doesn't matter… right!? Again, gems and stones can be purchased online, in specialty and department stores (at Tiffany's, of course!)… but do not discount the romance and personal history of *borrowed* and/or *heirloom* gems and stones for their symbolism, significance, or magic!

CHALCEDONY

A translucent gem of the quartz family, this stone is often smoky blue... but chalcedony also comes in white and yellow. Its magical properties include: creating balance in the body, mind, and spirit (let's face it, just what we need during this time!); eliminating irritability; and increasing responsiveness (*sexual* in this case, guys)! And as a touch of magic, chalcedony is reputed to increase the supply of mother's milk... just for some *future* reference, ladies!

CHRYSOPRASE

A green form of chalcedony... the color giving it its fertility powers... chrysoprase stimulates physical energy and love energy, and also increases dexterity... yes, dexterity! You may want to go immediately to Chapter 14 - SEX!

EMERALD

The green color of emerald alone is symbolic of fertility, but this stone goes far beyond its color in its powers to bring successful love, ensure domestic tranquility, stimulate the heart, arouse deep awareness, and bring good fortune. What more could you ask for in preparation for a baby!?... except perhaps a trip to the Emerald Isle!?

GARNET

Any stone that increases circulation to the pelvic area may just be the stone for you and your husband! And if that's not powerful enough... garnet also enhances sexual stimulation and fertility. Known as the stone of commitment and passion... garnet vitalizes, strengthens, energizes, and rejuvenates! Use with abandon! And if you want to get a little wild, as a touch of magic, place a garnet over your uterus and ovaries to not only reduce menstrual pain, but to restore physical strength. Oh, yes!

MOONSTONE

A cloudy, white, feldspar stone... moonstone is said to hold an image of the actual moon! Lovers have long revered moonstone for its power to enhance passion... and for your purposes, moonstone also promotes fertility! So use moonstone to *glow* all night long!

PEARL

Considered feminine, a pearl is a product of the oyster (remember, nature's finest aphrodisiac!), and can come from either sea water or fresh water. Pearls may range in color from white to black... but are commonly pale and shimmery. The magical properties of pearls bring wonders - peace of mind, focus, wisdom, patience, love, gentleness, and protection... all properties that are important in the pearl's finest magic - fertility! Legend has it that pearls are so closely related to fertility because of the time, patience, and yes, even miracle, that it takes for one oyster to produce even one pearl... just like the time and patience and miracle it takes to create even one baby!

QUARTZ - Clear and Rose

Clear - We'll give you a touch of magic about clear quartz first... if you hold clear quartz at your solar plexus and steady your breathing for several minutes, your body will relax, your mind will clear, your emotions will be calmed, and your energy will surge! Need we say more!?

Rose - Known as the *love stone*, rose quartz stimulates both the heart and the blood, and consequently stimulates *other* organs as well! And if that's not enough, rose quartz is known to stimulate sexual energy and to enhance fertility. Just think... all this power in a little stone! So place one (or more!) on your body, near your body, in your bedroom... or anywhere that the two of you meet... for delicious intimacy or passionate love-making!

RUBY

Generally red in color... ruby is the gemstone of power and passion. Its properties range from stimulating love and emotions, to promoting mental concentration. The ruby also protects the wearer against unhappiness... and is even reputed to prevent miscarriage. Because good spirits are said to dwell in the stone, it is no coincidence that all Dorothy had to do was click her *ruby* slippers in order to return to the safety and love of her home. So to maintain the joy, passion, and love at home... bring on the ruby!

~

OK, so back to diamonds! Although not a traditional lust or fertility gem, the diamond possesses the magic properties of permanence, fidelity, strength, and protection - four important and powerful qualities when thinking of multiplying your love by conceiving a child. So when all is said and done, maybe diamonds really *are* a girl's best friend!

We also just want you to keep in mind that there are hundreds of gems, stones, and precious metals that are rich in symbolic representations... and different sources site different magical properties for the same gems. Our list is comprised of the more common gems and stones consistently cited as love, lust, or fertility enhancers. But remember... don't trade in Grandma's heirloom jewelry if its not on our list - wear it because of the powers of family, of tradition, and of love. A child will come from this magic!

CHAPTER 12

Dance & Music

And we should consider every day lost on which we have not danced at least once.

- *FRIEDRICH NIETZSCHE*

You all have your own song that gets you moving… tapping your feet… performing in front of your mirror (come on, you know you've done it!)… blowing or strumming your air instrument… singing alone in the car or shower… or a song that reminds you of your lover. This is nothing new! We've all been *center stage* to an audience of one!

Since man first found a round hollow object, stretched some sort of skin over it, and grabbed two sticks with which to drum (hmm… sounds exotic!)… music and dance have enriched our lives every day, in every way, particularly involving sex and fertility.

Just think, from the time puberty kicked in… dances, proms, mixers, and parties probably became the focus of your teenage years. This is no coincidence, for music and dance - the rhythm and motion - are the powerful forces, some believe divinely created, to bring women and men nearer to their instinctive natures to mate - and yes, we bet you never thought of that, huh!?

And let's just be honest - with the *right* person and the *right* music... because, after all, maybe jazz gets your body willing to surrender to the passion of love (or country, classical, rock - soft or hard [pun intended], rap, soul, blues, or even Gregorian Chant!... you get the idea) - it's all about freedom, touch, passion, rhythm, and relaxation... all sensuously combined to enhance the mood for delicious sex!

So let us entertain you with some *fertility dance* tidbits, as well as some fertility dances, said to not only awaken your deepest sexuality, but also to increase and improve the task of, and the grade, rank, character, and nobility of... yes, the "little swimmers"... your husband's sperm!

So to make your sex even more enhanced...
You may just want to sing and dance!

Fertility dances have always been ritualistic in nature, sacred to the people, and performed to propagate clans. Surprise! Surprise! Surprise! Not much has changed! We still sing about sex. We still dance sexy dances. But what we need to keep in mind is that we are following the sacred sex and fertility rites of all of our ancestors. The universality of these dances and songs is what will... hopefully... make your baby-making even more sexy and significant and honorable. Because... after all, people have been sensuously singing and dancing forever!

Perform these at your own "risk"!

THE VOLTA

Think high voltage! Think intensity! Think electrical! Think excitement! Grab what we'll call a *twirling skirt*... a skirt that twirls perpendicular to your body as you spin. These skirts have been used as fertility costumes in multiple cultures just about forever... for the exposing of the female legs as she dances, and the flirtatious nature of the twirling skirt, both communicate the powers of sexuality and fertility. And for those of you who may not want your legs exposed up to, and possibly beyond your derriere, the Minuet dance will do! As a more refined form of The Volta, the Minuet still includes the lifting of your skirt in a sexy, but very *dainty* manner. Either of these dances will kick up your passion a few *volt*-as!

HOOTCHIE KOOTCHIE

The name alone conjures up a feeling of release and wild abandonment! Just say it - *Hootchie Kootchie*! This dance itself was introduced at the Chicago World's Fair in 1893 in all of its shocking, delicious sexiness; but in fact, the *Hootchie Kootchie* is a form of what is known as an "abdominal dance" (or some call "belly dance")! Abdominal dances, dating back to primitive man as fertility dances, involve movements of the pelvic region - you know... the thrusting, the rhythm, the rocking and the rolling of the entire pelvic area, the circular motion purposely indicative of the "circle of life"! Just think about it... the movements simulate the sexual act; and further, as a beautiful baby-making tidbit, many cultures performed abdominal dances as a "magical" way to promote fertility (of course it did!... as we know today that the movements of the pelvic region stimulate blood flow to the all-important reproductive areas!). So come on... choreograph your own Hootchie Kootchie to your favorite music! Your husband will love you for it! And remember, the less clothing, the better!

And while we're talking about pelvic moves... why not **leap** to...

LEAP DANCE!

Close the shutters... pull the shades... draw the curtains! You may not want your neighbors to see you perform this one! Leap dances incorporate both leaps (of course!) and interestingly enough, high kicks… as both **leaps** and **kicks** require a great deal of energy and vitality. It is energy and vitality and the ability to perform these dances that express the powers of the body and its reproductive force. Originally, it seems that primitive cultures used leap dances as *crop* fertility enhancers. As legend has it, as high as the leaper could leap was as high as the leaper's crops would grow! Hmmm… but the custom gradually changed in that the male would display his *physical* stamina, virility, and capabilities to his woman with his *talented* leaps and kicks, thereby turning the Leap Dance into a *human* fertility rite. So… for the guys… just how **long** and **high** can you go!?

And for you ladies, fortunately you're *not* off the hook! An interpretation of the Leap Dance, introduced in Paris in 1830, is the *Can-Can Dance*… which features high kicks, lifting of the skirts, and kicking off the hats of men in the audience. So… let's hope you're flexible! Hand your husband a hat and start kicking! Your performance should *kick in* enough stamina for both of you!

KAUSIMA

OK… you may want to send your husband on a 14-day sporting or business trip for this one! Indigenous to the South American Choroti Indian Tribe, the Kausima* is considered both a fertility dance and ritual, as well as a puberty rite-of-passage. In order to do this at home, you will need your mother and a group of older women (and yes, preferably women you know quite well!)… and (memorize your Moon Phases, see page 193!) these women must all arrive at the New Moon and stay until the Full Moon! First, you must stand motionless against any wall in your home. Next, the group of women must slowly circle your home, chanting (well, we're not sure what… perhaps, "Let's hope this works!") while pounding *Kahuis* on the ground. These Kahuis, of course (and you may need to supply these!), are long, hollow, bamboo staffs with several deer hooves (yes, deer hooves) tied to the tops! The fertility magic comes from the fertility powers of the deer... and from the rhythm of the pounding of the staffs (*pounding* seems to work well in fertility rites)! Next step... get rid of the women and wait for your husband to return! After this experience, you may be willing to do just about anything to have him back! Yes... *anything*!

**The standard Kausima was performed at the first menstruation, so if it doesn't work - maybe you're just a little beyond puberty!*

In short, let's go back to what we've been saying all along... relaxation, fun, *awareness* of your body... *awareness* that you are not the center of the universe, but rather part of a miraculous whole... *awareness* of your deliciously sexy passion, and your desire to procreate because of the great love between you and your husband... *awareness* of the sounds, sights, movements, tastes, scents, and touches all around you... and *awareness* of the powerful sexual-fertility enhancers that people have recognized since the beginning of time! These awarenesses are what will enhance your preconception time... by focusing on the all-important *just relaxing* part of the process, and enjoying the deliciousness of it all!

Each dance that we mention in this **Dance and Music** chapter is intended to add fun, laughter, and vitality to your love-making. And let's face it, we're not really telling you anything new! 21st century man did not invent the concept that music leads to dance, dance often leads to passion, and passion creates magical love-making! So... go on, let loose and *dance*!

CHAPTER 13

Rituals, Blessings, & Journaling

There are many roads to happiness.

- *PINDAR*

Unless you come from a society or culture that performs rites of puberty... oh, such as being *heated* in a pit for three to ten days while your family sings songs and performs dances for you, or you were isolated with your grandmother for the length of your first menstruation while listening to sex advice, or during your first menstruation, you were instructed to pass special blessings into every object in your home... then you probably have not been formally initiated into the world of puberty, fertility, sex, and parenthood...

But you are reading this book!

And unless your husband, at the tender age of anywhere between twelve to fifteen was sent out on a vision quest, alone and naked in the middle of the winter, with nothing but his bow and arrow, and told to come back with some animal that would feed his entire tribe... or at the very least instructed to stay in the wilderness until he had communicated with some supernatural spirit… then he has not been formally initiated into the world of puberty, fertility, sex, and parenthood…

But he, too, is reading this book (at least the Red-Flagged sections)!

It is interesting to note that primitive cultures marked the passage from childhood to adulthood… the time when a young woman began to menstruate, and therefore was capable of conceiving a child… through specific puberty rituals; and at approximately the same age for young men (ages twelve to fifteen), puberty rituals were also performed. Sometimes we may laugh at these ancient rituals (we mean, talking to your grandmother about sexual positions and multiple orgasms!?)… yet oddly enough, in all of our sophistication, it is our modern western culture that has a void in this area. As a society, we celebrate ourselves and our children with ceremonies surrounding birth, entry into a religious community, marriage, and death. We could say that a Confirmation, or a Bar/Bat Mitzfah, or even high school graduation is indeed our rite-of-passage into adulthood… but do any of these ceremonies truly prepare us, like primitive cultures prepared their adolescents, for the irrevocable split from childhood into the world of ripe sex, fertility, and parenthood!?

Ancient cultures of people knew how imperative it was to prepare their young adults for fertility, sex, and parenthood… and even further, their ceremonies most often involved the entire tribe or society, for young adults who were not prepared for the endurance, dedication, and knowledge of fertility, sex, and parenthood would be considered a detriment to the culture itself!

But you and your husband are on your own journey to prepare physically, emotionally, psychologically, and spiritually for fertility, sex, and parenthood! So possibly allow the ceremonies of **rituals, blessings**, and/or **journaling** to fit into your preconception journey!

Creating Your Own Rituals

Simply put, rituals are ways to get us in touch with a life-change, an affirmation, or an intention. In simpler terms, do you recite a prayer, or prayers, before bedtime? Do you use journals or diaries to collect your daily thoughts? Do you call your mother-in-law every Sunday (or do you remind your husband to do so)? Do you and your husband have a special (all cell phones off) Friday night date night? Believe it or not, these are rituals that we build into our lives... some simple, some more complex, some requiring little thought, some requiring more preparation.

Because rituals focus us and encourage us to enter into states of peace and comfort, it seems only natural that you may wish to adopt special rituals in preparing yourselves for conception (or, maybe not)! But in either case, here are some suggestions! And we promise, we won't be asking you to send your naked husband out into the wilderness (unless, of course, he wants to)!

So to send your positive energy into the air...
Rely on rituals, blessings, and prayers!

THE SUPER-EASY RITUALS

You've already read about foods... flowers... oils... herbs... scents... colors... candles... stones and gems... dance and music. The good news is, you can easily incorporate any or all of these into your own special fertility rituals!

How!? Well, since rituals force you to concentrate on your intention(s), while simultaneously bringing a sense of peace and structure to your life, why not light a red or green candle every night at dinner? Perhaps shower (or bathe) with your husband every Saturday morning? Enjoy a deliciously sexy aphrodisical dinner during your ovulation time? Select one night each week for some deliciously sensual dancing? Or choose one day each week to replace or refresh your cut flowers... come on, guys, this is why we call these *Super Easy Rituals*! Perhaps, for one deliciously sexy ritual, choose Wednesday (the "hump" day – pun intended) to try a new sexual position! And, if all else fails, invite your grandmother over once a week for sex advice!

The possibilities are endless... and this is just how easy it is to design and implement your own special rituals during your preconception time!

Blessings and Prayers

Blessings and prayers, sometimes associated with rituals (religious services, prayer before bed, grace before meals, etc.), are expressions of faith, focus, and belief... sometimes called **positive energy**. Blessings and prayers also capture dreams, and turn them into energy. Some people call this communication with God, some people call this visualization... but whatever your beliefs, the manner in which you precondition your mind is of vital importance. Preconditioning, whether through prayers or blessings or visualization, tends to create reality. Whatever you picture *about* yourself, or *for* yourself... *and the manner in which you truly believe it will come true*... simply ignites an inner and outer confidence.

Prayer is such a personal dialogue - here we offer an overview:

TIDBIT According to findings published in the ***Journal of Reproductive Medicine*** (October 2, 2001), a group of women undergoing in-vitro fertilization procedures had a 50% pregnancy rate when people prayed for them, as opposed to a 26% pregnancy rate in women who did not have people praying for them!

WHO PRAYS?

Some blessings and prayers will involve just you... some will incorporate your husband... some may be addressed by your family, friends, and beyond. In other words, you and your husband may consider your baby discussions to be very personal expressions to each other only, or perhaps to a higher being; but, if you've made the decision to share the news that you're thinking of having a baby, you may want the power of *collective communication* to ask for this blessed event!

WHAT DO YOU PRAY FOR?

This is as individual and as sacred as your marriage. Some people pray to get pregnant immediately. Some people pray to leave the decision in the hands of a higher power ("if it happens, it happens"). Some people are specific enough to pray for either a boy or a girl! Some even pray for multiple births – just to kind of "get it all done in one shot" (pun intended)! And most people pray for the blessing of a "healthy" baby!

WHY DO YOU PRAY?

It is focus… focus… focus! It is faith… faith… faith! It is preparation… preparation… preparation! And it is belief… belief… belief that you, and all of the elements in your life – physical, emotional, psychological, and spiritual – are bursting to multiply!

WHERE TO PRAY?

People pray everywhere! In the car… in bed… in the shower… at their desks (of course, on your down time!)… while exercising… or resting… while doing housework… and, of course, at religious services. The point is, *anywhere* at *anytime*. But some people feel a greater connection to a higher power if there is a symbol of prayer involved – an altar, a sacred space, an object, or even a gesture.

AN ALTAR OR SACRED SPACE

An altar or sacred space can be anywhere that makes you feel whole, happy, and calm. These personal spaces may simply be a shelf, a windowsill, a mantel, a corner of your desk, an entire room, a hatbox, a drawer... or even a space on your kitchen counter! The altar or sacred space becomes energized by the special symbols or objects that you place on it, or in it - perhaps special photographs, fertility amulets, your favorite flowers in a beautiful vase, or a religious symbol that is dear to your heart. Just think of things that bring to you a sense of togetherness, love, joy, affirmation, and fertility. Be imaginative! Be silly! Be sentimental! This is your special space to dream, to think, to love, to pray, and to be.

GESTURES

By gestures, we mean holding hands or blowing kisses or kneeling at an altar - or perhaps even *thumbs up* or *breasts up*! - gestures that simply reinforce the energy that turns your wishes into realities!

OBJECTS

Yet again, objects tend to focus our strength, our spirit, and our vitality – simply because they are visual, concrete reminders of our wishes! Any reminder is yet another positive affirmation of the direction of our energy.

WHEN TO PRAY?

Any time, anywhere... alone, or with anyone with whom you share a special bond!

Journaling

Journal writing is something that you will either do religiously, or something that you probably will not do at all. We're just being honest. But whether you do or do not, journaling is not some project designed by your 7th grade English teacher, comprised of various "thought" questions, and then graded! Journaling is intended to not only chronicle your days and your thoughts, but to release and focus and *make whole* your feelings, hopes, dreams, goals, wishes, intentions... and even disappointments and losses. Honest journaling allows you to *see* your growth and wisdom as an individual.

Since you are in the process of thinking about, or perhaps talking about, conceiving a baby... what more precious gift could you give to your child (some 15 to 20 years from now!) than the journey* to *have* that very child (and yes, we *will* say that a daughter may appreciate this gift more than a son)!

And further still, your *journal* may become your object or symbol of *fertility*... and the actual act of journaling may become your own special *ritual*!

**Point of warning! Your child will have no interest in reading about the delicious sex that you performed on the journey to conception.*
Keep that journal (or video!) separate and, well... locked!

CHAPTER 14

Sex

The nearer the bone, the sweeter the meat.

- *Portuguese Proverb*

Sex! This may just be the chapter you've been waiting for… (and ladies, if the pages are a bit tattered – perhaps your husband has already been here!); unless, of course, this is the first chapter you've flipped to!

And before we even get going, we do want you to remember that we assume you are in the preconception mode… where knowledge, facts, fun, and delicious sex in *preparation for conception* are key!

All right… so let's get down-and-dirty! There's probably a condom or diaphragm still in use… but your birth control pills, your IUD, or your patch is history, or almost history! Sex at this time, while preparing yourself for pregnancy, can be as highly seductive, as extremely sensuous, and as intensely passionate and intimate as sex for conception!

Intimacy right now is truly between just the two of you… no worrying yet if *it worked*, not yet fully consumed with *day 14*, while at the same time with no real nervousness if anything should happen to rip or tear or break or slip. This is the time when you get to concentrate on pleasing each other, or experimenting with each other… not necessarily trying to create a baby (yet)!

This is *sex*! This is love-making! Be wild! Shift your intimacy up a notch! Flirt with each other! Light candles! Strip-tease and dance naked! Consume foods and drinks rich in aphrodisical properties! Massage each other with essential oils! Take a "lunch" break! Buy each other a special fertility amulet! Purchase crisp, new sheets and scent them with your favorite fertility aroma! Add flowers! Write love notes to each other! Recite love poems! Shower together! Bathe together! And as a touch of magic... whip up a little Eros Oil to further enhance the mood! Simply mix 3 drops of Lavender Oil, 3 drops of Orange Oil, and 1 drop of Lemon Oil... and rub this mixture onto a candle of your choice (preferably red, green, or white!) and allow enough time for some... ohh... deliciously simple foreplay and deliciously sexy sex!

Feel the power, strength, vitality, and virility of your bodies. Keep in mind that most cultures and religions celebrate the concept that a man and a woman are not complete until they, in effect, share a single body... and this happens only when a man and a woman are *unified* - physically, emotionally, and spiritually - in the actual act of love-making.

OLD WIVES' TALE: If you want a **girl**... initiate sex, use the missionary position, and make sure that you have an orgasm first! If you want a **boy**... try making love standing up, sleep to the left of your husband, and make sure that your husband has an orgasm first!

Know that for the next month or two... or three or six or ten (or for however long you choose to prepare), you will experience each other in the most deliciously sexy ways imaginable! What wonderful and loving preparation for your future child!

And no matter what your preference or pleasure in sexual

positions, we're going to offer to you the recommended "not-so-best" as well as the "best" positions for making babies! So start practicing! Become very, very familiar with these positions, so that when you are ready for baby-making, you are already relaxed and absolutely loving it!

So get reading… and let's hope you can make it to the end of this chapter!

**When making a baby becomes your *mission*…
Perfect your talents with these sexual positions!**

"Not-So-Best!" Positions

In case you are straddling your husband while reading this book - hop off right now! The rule of thumb (or whatever index we're discussing) is that any position that makes the sperm swim *upward* should be *avoided* (for baby-making purposes) at all costs! We guess that most sperm don't want to work that hard! Let's face it… if you're sitting *on* your husband, gravity is going to pull the sperm back downward (leakage), rather than towards your cervix. After all, *the starting line is your cervix*, so you should do everything possible to help the little swimmers *win*!

And while we're on the subject of upward swimming sperm, if sex while standing or sitting is your "thing"… well, sprawl, repose, recline, be supine… bottom line, just *lie down* if conception is your immediate aim!

"Best" Positions

Man on top! This is, hands down (or at least *your back down*!) the absolute, most highly recommended, across-the-board-best-sexual-position for making babies! The best! And this may not even come as a surprise to you! We mean, just think about it… with the man on top, the missionary position provides deeper penetration (which we're not complaining about!), and the sperm, once ejaculated, swim *downstream*... making the race to the cervix much more probable.

And for the ladies... another baby-making tip! Remain on your back after love-making, but place a pillow under your pelvic area and stay this way for about a half an hour. This may sound like an Old Wives' Tale... but in reality, this allows the sperm some additional time to travel, perhaps even reaching as far as your fallopian tubes. Some women also swear by the *bicycle motion* at this time to further help the sperm reach their goal!

> **TIDBIT** This may be a wild one (and a bit unsanitary for our tastes!)... but right before love-making, egg whites (yes... egg whites!) applied to your husband's penis are reputed to not only help the sperm travel quickly, but help them to stay alive longer as well! Seems that the calcium content in egg whites is very sperm-friendly!

And for the guys, you may **not** want to grab the remote, get a beer, pull out the sports page, call your mother, or tell her about your busy day (and never go near the "what you can't afford" line after love-making)! Instead, take this gift of time... as your baby may be in the making... and just talk and laugh and talk and laugh. Think positive here... at the end of the thirty minutes of pelvic-pillow-time, you and she may just get lucky again! All this talking and laughing (and "cycling") may lead to even more deliciously sexy sex!

And keep in mind that, yes, you can be very creative with the missionary-style position. There's always the "leg lock" or "shoulder lock"! And even though we're pretty sure that you can figure out how to do these on your own, or at least your own variations, we're not going to just leave you hanging!

> **TIDBIT** It seems that the morning is the best time to have *conception* sex, for a man's sperm count is at its highest. So lucky you! Who needs coffee?

THE "LEG LOCK"

The Leg Lock simply requires that you "lock" your legs around your husband's body. Pretty good, huh!? What this position does is to allow for deeper penetration... and therefore gives the sperm more of a head start!

THE "SHOULDER LOCK"

The Shoulder Lock is quite simple to explain, but really could depend upon your own flexibility! Intrigued already? Just place your legs on your husband's shoulders, one leg on each side of his head. The farther back your legs go, the deeper the penetration into your vagina! Let's just hope you're into yoga, or that you are an ex-gymnast!

SIDE-BY-SIDE POSITION

This position is exactly what its name suggests – partners face-to-face, lying down side-by-side. This position prevents leakage of sperm... and is highly recommended for people who may have a hard time with the missionary position due to weight problems, or muscle or back related problems. Just keep thinking... the good news about this position is that the sperm swim straight *in*, not *up*!

> **TIDBIT** www.elevatedconceptions.com recommends Liberator® Shapes™ – the Wedge™, the Ramp™, the Stage™, and the Cube™ to enhance love-making and conception! According to its web page, you'll be "rocking, tilting, inclining, bouncing, and best of all... conceiving!"

REAR-ENTRY POSITION

And we're talking into the *vagina*! For conception purposes, this position is recommended in either the kneeling or lying down position (ooh-lah-lah!). In this way, leakage of sperm is prevented... and at the risk of sounding repetitive, it should be a *straight shot* to the cervix!

And don't forget... that even with the Side-by-Side Position and the Rear-Entry Position, take the time to do the thirty-minute pillow talk! Hey... anything that may help is worth trying!

Although you and your husband may or may not be familiar with the recommended conception sex positions... as we suggest here... *practice*! You may find that it takes a little time to release your inhibitions, get comfortable with certain positions, or just simply, and most importantly... *enjoy them*!

And while we're on the subject of enjoyment... let's talk orgasms! We all know that a man *must* ejaculate in order to conceive a baby (and yes, we are all familiar with the story of someone who knows someone who got pregnant with the pre-ejaculate – but we're talking the norm...), but let's talk about you, a *woman*! Obviously, female orgasms are not prerequisites for conception... but some studies indicate that a female orgasm creates a series of contractions that further aid the sperms' journey into the cervix. This is precisely why we're encouraging you to practice the "best" conception positions... because most women need to feel uninhibited and comfortable with sex before it can truly be enjoyed to the height of orgasm!

But please do not get hung up on, "We must do *this* position, Honey!" or "I must have an orgasm, Honey!" (though we'd all like to)! Baby-making is about *relaxing* – and let's be honest... if you're relaxed and comfortable, the intimacy and passion will lead to orgasm.

Enjoy sex! Enjoy each other! Enjoy the different positions we've mentioned. Allow your love and your passion to make *every* time you're together absolutely exhilarating!

OLD WIVES' TALE: More babies are born on October 5th than any other calendar date... count back to possible date of conception – New Year's Eve!

CHAPTER 15

Fertility Spells & Wishes

Events, circumstances, have their origin in ourselves.
They spring from seeds that we have sown.
- HENRY DAVID THOREAU

Difficult to really define, *magic* is a touch of the unknown... a leap of faith... sometimes referred to as wish power... maybe even an enchanted world in which you have never stepped? Well, why not be a little bold... a little brave... and yes, even a little ballsy! Fun, intriguingly simple, and downright deliciously sexy, *magic* is positive thinking... a child-like faith in the finest gifts that the universe has to offer! Uncover this newness in your quest for a child. Remember that spells*, prayers, and rituals are all faith-based, concentrated energies that are available for us to call upon in our lives.

And... please may it be known that we are by no means experts in this field! But we were given the most exquisitely honest advice from a witch in Salem, Massachusetts, who explained to us, "Why fight with the universe when you can simply work with the universe." Well said!

If you think of a *spell* as a fascinating charm or verse... an enthralling power... or mystical fun – you're going to love these fabulously-fun, fertility-focused, even folklorish spells! You will discover in the following spells and wishes that the needed ingredients are easily attainable… and the words of the spells effectively beautiful.

And now… keeping in mind that you are in the preconception stage, with the hopes of conception in the future (near or otherwise), we encourage you, as with everything else in this book, to familiarize yourself with these fertility spells *before* actually casting them… and amend the ingredients and/or words as needed in order to express your own passions and creativity! These are spells… both ancient and modern… created specifically for conception.

So ponder, prepare, and practice your spells…
For what the magical future tells!

**Read each spell very carefully before performing… as some are rather specific in terms of time and need!*

Fertility Spells!

SPELL #1... To be performed any time!

INGREDIENTS:

Your voices!
Your wishes!

To each direction – North, South, East, West – recite the following with love and conviction:

To you, my child, my body is open.
To you, my child, my mind is open.
To you, my child, my heart is open.
By Earth, Fire, Wind and Sea-
Into my arms you will be.

The last two lines are recited while gazing upon your own cradled arms.

SPELL #2... To be performed during OVULATION!

INGREDIENTS:

Apple Scented Cream or Lotion
A String of Pearls - Pearls need not be real...
unless you tell your husband that it's necessary!

Remember that both apples and pearls are powerful fertility symbols!

After a relaxing shower or bath... massage your body (or preferably have your husband massage your body) with the Apple Scented Cream or Lotion, taking care to give special attention to your abdomen. Imagine warmth... a glowing golden warmth that fills your abdominal area. Strongly and lovingly visualize that conception is very possible while you or your husband clasp the string of Pearls around your neck, as you confidently recite:

> Precious jewels of Lunar,
> I offer this adornment.
> In honor of your power, let fertile light shine through me.
> Blessed be.

SPELL #3... To be performed with your husband in an Easterly Wind, representing new beginnings!

INGREDIENTS:

- 14 Nuts*
- 14 Seeds*
- 2 Pieces of Green Cloth (*green* representing *growth*)
  Make sure the cloth is large enough to bundle 7 seeds and 7 nuts!
- 2 Yellow Ribbons (*yellow* representing *creativity*)
  Make sure the ribbon is long enough to tie around the cloth bundles!

> **TIDBIT** Kwan Yin is the Chinese Goddess of Fertility, called *she who brings children...* and she is often depicted with a child in her arms. Kwan Yin has been known to grant pregnancy to those who place embroidered slippers before her image!

Both you and your husband must gather 7 nuts and 7 seeds each (*gather your favorites... but preferably from our list of fertility nuts and seeds, see page 106)! In an Easterly wind... each of you must bundle your own nuts and seeds in your green cloth, and each of you must then tie your bundle with your yellow ribbon, and knot your ribbon 7 times. With each knot, recite the following:

Kwan Yin, see our hearts.
To our bodies, your blessings impart.
Fill these tokens with fertility;
And let our love manifest in pregnancy.

Carry your bundles in your pockets, or close to your hearts, whenever possible; but during delicious sex… make sure to keep one bundle on each side of your bed for that positive energy to surge and vitalize!

Adapted from "Conception Charm", **Goddess In My Pocket,** *by Patricia Telesco.*

SPELL #4… Perform during the Waxing to Full Moon! (see page 193 for Moon Phases)

INGREDIENTS:

1 Egg
1 Drinking Straw
Small Sheet of Clean Paper
Writing Utensil or Marker
Soft Fabric of your choice for a Makeshift Cradle

OK, this may not be the easiest thing to do, but it sure is fun to try!

You must hollow an egg by blowing out the yolk and the white. This may take a few tries before you actually get it right… but we can guarantee that this part of the spell will bring some laughter… some memories… or maybe even a new skill! But let's go back to the beginning… first, hollow out an egg!

After hollowing, decorate your egg – very carefully – using any symbols or words or images that, to you, best represent being pregnant. On the sheet of paper, write your wish for a baby… and then delicately roll and insert this note into the shell of your egg (you may have to roll your note tightly to get it in)!

Place your egg in the light of a Waxing to Full Moon (see page 193) for three nights… then place it in your fabric cradle and place the cradle near your bed. Let your egg remain there until the next Waxing to Full Moon… or when you know you are ovulating. Stand before the egg, place your hands over it, and allow the energy of this fertility symbol and your loving wishes to become as full as the growing moon. "A little complicated!" you may think?… but definitely worth the time, fun, effort, togetherness, and energy that this spell will bring!

Adapted from "Eggs-actly!", **Goddess In My Pocket,** *by Patricia Telesco.*

SPELL #5… To Conceive A Son!… Perform during Ovulation!

INGREDIENTS:

- 1 Red Rose
- 1 Vase
- 1 Red Candle
- 1 Green Candle
- 1 Yellow Candle
- 1 Bay Leaf
- 1 Pen/Marker

At your most fertile time of the month, place one red rose in a vase on a table. Light a red candle, which is symbolic of Mars, ruler of vigor and vitality. Next, light a green candle. This color is associated with Venus, love, and harmony. Place it to the right of the red candle. Place a yellow candle, to represent the sun, above the red and green candles to form a triangle. The number three represents the male reproductive organs, and sexual force.

On a bay leaf - because bay is ruled by the sun - write the phrase "I wish to conceive a son." Place it face up between the candles.

Now close your eyes and imagine a red rosebud in your womb. Visualize the rosebud unfolding and coming into bloom.

Open your eyes and visualize the candlelight being channeled into your womb, then close your eyes and continue with the visualization for as long as you can.

Leave the candles to burn themselves out. Take the bay leaf, kiss it three times, and place it under your pillow, where it should stay throughout your fertile phase.

All that is required now is the cooperation of your partner.

The Good Spell Book, *by Gillian Kemp.*

SPELL #6... To Conceive A Daughter!... To Be Performed When You Are Approaching Ovulation!

The purpose of this spell is to make a doll that resembles you... seem difficult?... not really, if you allow your imagination and creativity to kick in! So here goes...

INGREDIENTS:

Modeling Clay
A Snip of Your Hair
Small Clothing or Fabric
Photograph of Your Face
Fresh Lavender or Pink Scarf, Sprayed with Lavender Oil
1 Small Pink Candle
1 Sheet of Clean, White Paper
1 Piece of Yellow Ribbon
1 Quartz Crystal
1 Moonstone

You need to prepare and work this spell when you are reaching your most fertile time of the month.

The idea is to make a doll that resembles you as closely as possible. Take some modeling clay and mold it into the form of a pregnant woman; press hair from your comb into her head, dress her in clothes like yours, even cut out a photo of your face and place it on hers.

When the doll is prepared, place her on a bed of fresh lavender or on a pink scarf sprinkled with lavender oil (lavender is a masculine flower, as its shape dictates, and it attracts love). Take her to a table in a room without electric lights, and light a pink candle to the right of her.

Using clean white paper, write the phrase "I wish to conceive a daughter". Place the paper beneath the lavender or scarf.

Fold the paper around the doll on her bed and tie a yellow ribbon or cord around her. Place your doll beside your pillow, or on a bedside table, with a piece of Quartz Crystal and a Moonstone. Quartz is sometimes called "sacred fire" because it intensifies the rays and energy of the sun, a masculine force. Moonstone, governed by the moon, is a feminine, emotional stone. Its nature and aura improve health and reveal the future. Like females, it changes with the moon: it transmits energy to health when the moon is waxing and gives power to desires when the moon is waning.

Your partner's desire completes the spell and brings it to fruition.

The Good Spell Book, *by Gillian Kemp.*

Wishes!

WISHES COME TRUE #1...

To be performed on the Night of a New Moon (see page 193)!

INGREDIENTS:

1 Bay Leaf
1 Pen/Marker
Confidence!

On the night of a New Moon, write your wish on the bay leaf. Simply take the bay leaf outside and look at the Moon, then kiss the bay leaf three times and sleep with this bay leaf under your pillow.

Since the bay tree is governed by the sun and ruled by Leo, this charm is particularly potent when the sun is in Leo, between July 23 and August 22.

WISHES COME TRUE #2... To be Performed at Any Time!

INGREDIENTS:

Fresh St.-John's-wort
1 Small Orange Candle

TIDBIT: Candles should always be allowed to extinguish themselves, or be snuffed... for *blown out* candles may *blow* your wishes away!

St.-John's-wort, a golden flower that smells like turpentine, is regarded as an emblem of the sun.

Light an orange candle and place a bunch of St.-John's-wort beside it. Make a wish, then hang the bunch of St.-John's-wort over an entrance door to your home. Leave the candle to extinguish itself. It will bring your wish and ward off evil too.

WISHES COME TRUE #3... To be Performed During the Night!

INGREDIENTS:

Night Sky, on any Night of the Year!
Faith on Your Part!

Wish upon the first star you see in the night sky, on any night of the year. Your wish will come true if a second star appears shortly afterward.

WISHES COME TRUE #4... To be performed on Halloween!

INGREDIENTS:

1 Pomegranate

On Halloween night, eat the seeds of a pomegranate as you make a wish for a child.

THE NEEDLE TRICK

INGREDIENTS:

1 Sewing Needle
1 Piece of Thread, Ribbon, or a Strand of Your Hair (at least 12 inches long)!

This is a fun game that you can try *before* you and your husband conceive, but definitely *after*!

Suspend a needle from your looped piece of thread, ribbon, or hair. Have your husband suspend the needle an inch above your hand. If the needle swings back and forth, a girl is in your future... .if it moves in a circular motion, a boy is in your future!

Spells for Brides!

If you desire children in either your near or far future!

SPELL #1... Rose Petal Path

Since the rose is recognized as the ultimate flower of love, it only seems natural that rose petals would find their way into marriage fertility rites! Rose petals not only grant fertility, but are reputed to guard against evil spirits... so spread rose petals along the aisles or pathways that you will walk upon as a newly married couple!

SPELL #2... Jumping Over the Broom

The broom is not only a symbol of cleansing at the beginning of your new life together, but also a powerful symbol of fertility... the handle (of course!) representing the masculine and the brush (oh, yes!) representing the feminine! You must jump over the broom (ask a very special person to purchase this broom for you!) as a married couple, in full wedding attire (whatever that may be!) on the day of your wedding. This rite/spell will bring children! And as a further touch of magic, leave your broom brush side up in your home to protect yourselves from negative energies!

SPELL #3... Egg Favor

Yes, it's that simple! You know by now that the egg is one of the most powerful of all fertility symbols... so incorporate eggs into your wedding rite by giving decorated eggs to your guests as favors. This is said to ensure fertility. So be creative... (and depending upon your budget)... these egg favors may be porcelain, glass, wax, wooden, plastic, terra cotta, crystal, even hard-boiled! As a touch of magic, your egg favors bring good fortune to whomever goes home with one!

CHAPTER 16

Moon Magic & Menstrual Magic

The day, water, sun, moon, night – I do not have to purchase these things with money.

- *PLAUTUS*

So... you may be wondering just how Moon Magic and Menstrual Magic fit into your delicious preconception time? Actually, it is very simple, it is very intriguing, and it will give you such beautiful knowledge of the phases that your own body experiences each month.

Whether you are planning to try to conceive next month, or even next year or beyond, awareness of the distinct phases of your menstrual cycle will relax you... and yes, may even *entertain* you (and your husband as well)!

And so... just how does the moon herself (yes, the moon is considered feminine in most cultures!) play a role in all of this? Well, just as the moon follows a $28\frac{1}{2}$ day cycle through its four important phases - New, Waxing, Full, Waning - each woman also has her own approximate $28\frac{1}{2}$ day (menstrual) cycle that brings her through her own four important phases. In ***Fertility Freedom***, Nadia MacLeod refers to these phases as

Virgin/Maiden... Mother/Empress... Enchantress... Crone.

The miracle in all of this is that the four phases of the moon cycle, and the four phases of the female menstrual cycle, mimic amazingly similar energies.

This is the key!

The reason you may want to know the nature of **moon/menstrual phases*** before you even try to conceive is so that you will understand and become aware of the natural energies of your own body. A marvelous bit of magic in all of this is that the universe experiences the same energies... making you a beautiful piece in all of this, rather than a separate part of it.

OLD WIVES' TALE: If you want a **boy**, make love when there is a quarter moon in the sky... have sex on *odd* days of the month... make sure your head is pointing north while having sex! If you want a **girl**, make love in the afternoon... have sex on *even* days of the month!

So Moons New, Waxing, Waning, or Full...
Think Beauty and Bounty and Power-ful!

Moon Cycle

NEW MOON

When there appears to be no moon in the sky... but, in fact, the moon is simply between the sun and the Earth and cannot reflect the sun's light. Margie Lapanja, author of ***The Goddess' Guide to Love***, describes the New Moon phase as *"a powerful and quiet night of reflection and re-dedication... a night to honor your desires."*

WAXING MOON

When the moon appears progressively more illuminated in the night sky… sometimes called the right-handed moon, as the curve of the crescent follows the curve of the right-hand index finger and thumb. As Margie Lapanja writes… *"a supercharged time of magic, fertility, and growth; a positive time for emanating energy of attraction, manifestation, and creation… begin new projects."*

FULL MOON

When the moon reaches her full illuminated capacity in the night sky… the sun and moon are opposite one another and the Earth is between them. According to Lapanja, this is *"the night to surrender to the passion of life and love; celebrate the fruits of your intentions."*

WANING MOON

When the moon appears progressively less illuminated in the night sky… sometimes called the left-handed moon, as the curve of the crescent follows the curve of the left-hand index finger and thumb. Lapanja describes this moon phase as *"a time to emit energy of release… diminishing, decreasing and dissipating."*

It is interesting to note that the words* **moon *and* **menses** *derive from the same word -* **measure***!*

Menstrual Cycle*

VIRGIN/MAIDEN

The term "Virgin" in this context is given to the ancient meaning of a woman who is fertile, sexual, and complete unto herself. It is a time to be bold, dynamic, energetic, confident, and "out there". A sociable and communicative time, where fresh starts, new projects and being in the physical world are the focus. There is new energy and a willingness to participate in the outer world in an independent and assertive manner. This time is self-aware, but with the desire to co-operate and interact with the world.

MOTHER/EMPRESS

Energy is ripe and full, just like the fertile egg at ovulation. We can nourish, nurture, sustain, and empower ourselves and our creative works. Receptivity, communion, and co-operation are highlighted, as we are ready to meet with and co-create with others. A time of focus on others with an enhanced ability to be self-sacrificing. Projects can be fertilized at this time, and it is often a good time to seek input from other beings (physical or spiritual) we trust.

ENCHANTRESS

An introspective time, we are drawn inwards to reflect on our place and progress in the world. We often need to be alone and can be intolerant of the demands put on us by others. We dream more, need more quiet time, are more intuitive, and can feel our sexuality peak, or take on a different flavor. The veil between the physical and spiritual world thins.

CRONE

Introspective and intuitive. Women are open to the messages

from the soul, about spiritual purpose, and what the individual requires to achieve happiness. A time of cleansing and release… as we let go of our blood during bleeding, we can let go of the thoughts, beliefs, and habits that do not serve us any longer. We can call on the "Crone" energy to destroy and remove anything we don't need any more. It is the seeding for the next cycle. Self-focused.

* *Source:* ***Fertility Freedom****, Nadia MacLeod, www.menstruation.com.au*

Magic Cycle

NEW MOON

Magical time of change…

WAXING MOON

Magical time of luck, love, and growth (the 3 days after the New Moon are the most powerful times to work spells for growth and beginnings, which come to fruition at the Full Moon)…

FULL MOON

Magical time of fertility, power, passion, knowledge, and dreams…

WANING MOON

Magical time of releasing the old, removing unwanted or negative energy…

As you can see from the **Moon/Menstrual/Magic Cycles**, and we must directly quote Nadia MacLeod here for she says it so eloquently, "Just as the moon waxes and wanes throughout the month, so do you. You experience different moods, desires and aspects of yourself (and being female) depending upon where you are in your menstrual cycle." And as you become more and more familiar with each menstrual phase, you will accept the sometimes subtle, and sometimes dramatic, changes in your body, your moods, and your needs.

Know yourself! Know that it's no coincidence that you are probably more sexually charged at the end of your Mother/Empress phase and the beginning of your Enchantress phase (ovulation) than you are in your Crone phase. Hey... at least now your husband can put nicknames to your *phases*... and better still, he will understand these phases as well as you do!

And for some touches of **Moon Magic**...

- If you make a wish upon seeing the **New Moon**... but keep the wish secret from everyone... it will come true!

- If you make a wish, and then kiss the nearest person to you upon seeing the **New Moon**, your wish will come true!

- **New Year Moons!** A wish spoken to the first New Moon of the New Year will be fulfilled. It is especially fortunate to see the New Moon Crescent on your right. The first Full Moon of the year is also said to make a wish come true, and your wish will be granted before the year is out.

- **Midsummer Night's Eve: June 20th!** To encourage good fortune... on Midsummer Night's Eve, take an orange (to represent the Sun) and a lemon (which symbolizes the Moon); press cloves (representing brown wooden nails) into the skin of the fruit. The cloves purge any misfortune that the first half of the year may have brought, and ensure that the second half of the year will be trouble free.

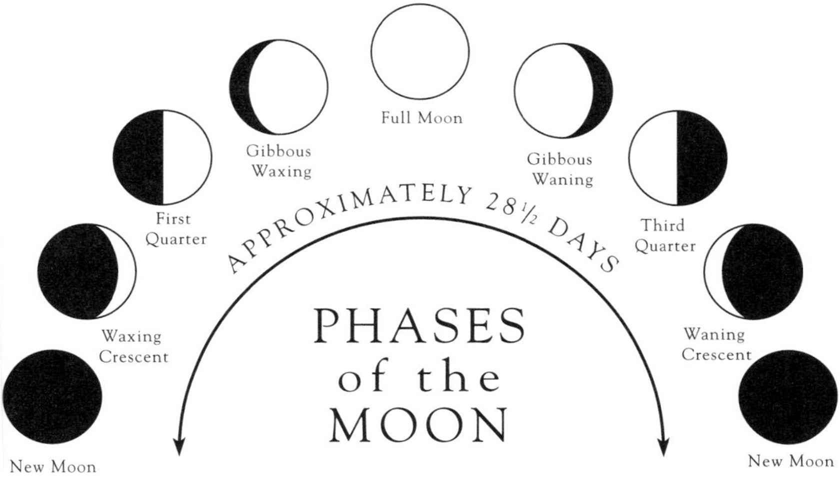

TIDBIT For more detailed moon information, visit:
http://www.shetline.com/java/moonphase/moonphase.html or
http://aa.usno.navy.mil/data/docs/MoonPhase.html

Just keep in mind that when you look to nature with belief and knowledge and affirmation, she will work with you. Again, it is no coincidence that we address nature as *Mother* in all of her nurturing splendor!

Believe!

Epilogue

He who is fixed to a star does not change his mind.

- Leonardo Da Vinci

Empowerment

As you know by now, our book ***Preconception Plain & Simple*** celebrates the very important tenets of unified focus… powerful affirmation… vital energy… and very conscious mindfulness of your physical health, emotional health, personal histories, and environment in your intention to conceive a child! In short, everything we mention in our book is *conception affirming* – a positive, consistent, and aligned convergence of intentions that unifies these fields of energy on all levels.

Now, of course, you and your husband will bring your own unified focus to your baby-making… whether it be through the medical component of getting your bodies ready for conception, dining on fertility foods, or perhaps through aromas, fertility symbols or amulets, music and dance, or incorporating prayers, blessings, journaling, or fertility spells and moon magic… any, or possibly all things that maintain a wonderfully consistent and high frequency of energy around your intention of conception!

Just remember that it is no coincidence that virtually every culture has its fertility gods and goddesses… fertility rituals and enhancers… fertility mythology… fertility dances… fertility/marriage rites… fertility foods… fertility gems and stones… a conscious seeking of just that affirmation – conception! It is no coincidence that peoples from all times and places have made mindful selections of objects and symbols, and the same mindful placement of objects and symbols… and yet again, mindful selections of blood-pumping dances and colors and scents and foods that not only optimally ready our bodies, but ready our environments as well for the desired result – conception! Now, again, some of you will choose as your focus the medical piece… readying your bodies for conception. Some of you will sort through **The Wings** and choose rituals, symbols, spaces, or faith-based traditions that create reminders of your readiness for conception. Others… (like me, Audrey!) will choose to do just about everything, perhaps for research, but more importantly, to activate and invigorate and engage all of your senses! But whatever you do choose, our message is one of positive focus, drawn from the knowledge and celebrations of so many… that vital energies will make you feel one with your intention!

And as much "smart" medical information as we now have at our fingertips regarding preconception and conception… well, it is simply not very fun, and it is not very sexy! Our hope is that ***Preconception Plain & Simple*** has given you a positive, heightened, non-fractured, and relaxed focus that allows you and your husband to create an **internal** (physical and emotional health/feelings!) preparation for conception that is beautifully aligned with your **external** (physical environment and actions!) preparation for conception!

Yes, your preconception and conception time will be **Smart, Fun & Sexy**!

AUDREY

While writing ***Preconception Plain & Simple,*** *what inspired me the most was dreaming about my future children. It was what fueled me to even begin writing this book with my mother… the passion that came from our hearts, our souls, our minds, and from my babies who would be!*

When my mother and I finished writing in December 2003, my husband and I knew that the time was right to start trying for our Little One. We had already been following all of the information and tidbits and recipes for the many months that I had been researching and writing… so, we thought, let's go for it!

Three weeks later, on January 17, 2004… at 9:08 am, our lives changed forever! There were ***two lines*** *on the pregnancy test! Two lines! I don't think any woman can possibly put into words the feeling that comes over her when she gets that positive confirmation… and I still get "goose bumps" when I think back to that very morning!*

My mother and I wrote our book with love and passion… and I followed the information in our book with the same love and passion… and most of all, my husband and I relaxed, had glorious fun, and deliciously sexy sex… and we loved each other more than is imaginable! This is the way we created our beautiful child!

As of this date, September 21, 2004, I am 39 weeks along in my pregnancy. We know we are having a boy! We do not know if our baby will be born on his due date… September 25, 2004. But what we do know is that this baby, the inspiration behind our book… was conceived by healthy parents, with wonderfully positive thoughts, some delectable aphrodisical foods, a little bit of "magic", and through prayer!

May we all have blessed, healthy, and beautiful babies!

Enjoy the ride!

SHARON

On the evening of January 5, 2004, I felt such an astounding warmth and beauty around me, that I felt compelled to write my thoughts… and these are the words that I wrote in my journal that night!:

January 5, 2004, 6:30 pm

To my sweet, sweet Grandchild…

I "feel" you all around me as I sit to write my very first thoughts of 2004!

I know you… have always known you… and I love

you with a love that has come over mountains and seas and oceans and deserts! I love you with the depth of every color that has ever existed, especially the soon-to-be-famous Pinks & Blues! I love you through my father and mother, who you will learn so much about... and through all generations whom have come before you in the minds, spirits, bodies, creativity, miracles, and courage of the Coutos and McClellands... the Klaczynskis and Bedzyks... and all of the countless others of Moms and Dads, Grandparents, Aunts and Uncles and Cousins whose biology you share!

I want, tonight, to tell you about your Mommy and Daddy! Of course, I have known your Mommy since before she was born... she, too, was once the "divine spark" that had to be "lit" by your Grandpa and me! Your Mommy... Audrey Couto McClelland, is the most beautiful, kind, compassionate, funny, loving "Mommy" who ever waited for a child! She has been talking about you for many, many years... as she has always been considered what some call an "old soul"!

This simply means that she believes, with fervent passion, that you have always been meant for her... and she has accomplished amazing things in her journey to have you! She has, for examples, fought to get into this world early... five full weeks early... shocking your Grandfather Couto and me – she has written beautiful words – she has swum countless races – she has traveled countless miles – she has met many, many people – she has been determined to succeed – all in preparation for meeting your Daddy... and then to have you! Your Mommy and Daddy have built a cozy nest in New York City, and they have surrounded it with greens and lavenders, herbs and spices, gems and stones... but more

importantly, they have filled their nest with such love… love that is at once miraculous and spiritual and passionate! Now they wait for you, their very first child… their dream made visible.

I think of you tonight… and I will think of you forever and ever and ever!

I will write tomorrow about your Grandpa Couto… the love of my life!

I love you already!
Grandma

The miracle in this process of writing and thinking and blessings and fertility and conception is that the passion of it all just pours out… and then comes back a million-fold! The baby "that would be", as Audrey writes, is the baby… my Grandchild… whom she and Matthew announced to my husband and me on the evening of January 17, 2004; and after the obstetrician visits and sonograms and calculations, the probable date of conception of this baby was - miraculously enough - January 5, 2004!

Belief in miracles… trust in God and saints and angels… passion of heart, soul, and mind… accepting the "gifts" that the universe has to offer… the blending of age and culture and religion and race and time… the journey of a mother and a daughter and womanhood… and now a Little One!

The cycle of life continues!

Believe!

Appendix

The following Lists appear in full detail:

Shopping List, *pages 89 - 110*
Preconception Examination Checklist, *pages 38 - 54*

Let's Get It On Shopping List

APPETIZERS

❑ ARTICHOKES

❑ CAVIAR

❑ CHEESE

❑ ENDIVE

❑ GUACAMOLE

❑ OYSTERS

MAIN DISHES

❑ BEEF

❑ SEAFOOD

❑ HOT DOGS

VEGETABLES

❑ ASPARAGUS

❑ CARROTS

❑ CELERY

❑ CHILI PEPPERS

❑ CUCUMBERS

❑ MUSHROOMS

❑ ONIONS

❑ RADISHES

❑ TOMATOES

❑ ZUCCHINI

ON THE SIDE

❑ RICE

❑ SWEET POTATOES

HERBS

❑ BASIL

❑ CAPERS

❑ DILL

❑ GARLIC

❑ PARSLEY

SPICES

❑ CINNAMON

❑ CLOVES

❑ GINGER

❑ NUTMEG

❑ PEPPER
Black, Green, or White

❑ SAFFRON

FRUITS

❑ APPLES

❑ APRICOTS

❑ BANANAS

❑ DATES

- ❑ FIGS
- ❑ GRAPES
- ❑ MANGOES
- ❑ MELONS
- ❑ OLIVES
- ❑ ORANGES
- ❑ PAPAYAS
- ❑ PEACHES
- ❑ PEARS
- ❑ STRAWBERRIES

CONDIMENTS

- ❑ HONEY
- ❑ MUSTARD

DESSERTS

- ❑ CHOCOLATE
- ❑ ECLAIRS
- ❑ LICORICE (Black)
- ❑ PUMPKIN PIE
- ❑ VANILLA

LATE NIGHT SNACKS

SEEDS AND NUTS

- ❑ CARAWAY
- ❑ CHESTNUT
- ❑ HAZELNUT
- ❑ PUMPKIN
- ❑ SESAME
- ❑ SUNFLOWER

BEVERAGES

- ❑ BEER
- ❑ CHAMPAGNE
- ❑ LEMON TEA
- ❑ LEMONADE
- ❑ MEAD
- ❑ MILK
- ❑ PEPPERMINT TEA
- ❑ SAKE
- ❑ SMOOTHIES
- ❑ TEQUILA
- ❑ WATER
- ❑ WINE

THE MORNING AFTER

- ❑ CAFFEINE
- ❑ CINNAMON BUNS
- ❑ DOUGHNUTS
- ❑ EGGS

Preconception Examination Checklist

GENERAL QUESTIONS/COMMENTS

My birth date is ______________________ (I am ___ years old).

My husband's birth date is ______________ (he is ___ years old).

This is our first time trying to conceive a baby ☐ yes ☐ no.

We plan to actively start trying ________________ (month/year).

We have been trying to conceive for ___ months/years.

The date of my last menstrual period was ____________________.

My periods are regular / irregular and come approximately every _________ days.

We are currently using _____________ as a birth control method.

I (we) have used (birth control methods) ____________, ___________, ________________ in the past.

Date(s): ____

I have been pregnant ____ times.

Date(s): ____

Weight of baby(ies): ____________________________________

Delivery Method(s): _____________________________________

Complications: ____

Premature births: _______________________________________

I have had ____ miscarriage(s).
Date(s): ______________________________

I have had ____ ectopic pregnancy(ies).
Date(s): ______________________________

I have had ____ abortion(s) - *(be sure to tell your physician where, when, and by whom, so that your physician will be able to determine if a pregnancy may be affected in any way)*.

My last Pap Smear was ____________________ (date).

My last Mammogram was ____________________ (date).

Can you recommend an excellent preconception/pre-natal woman's vitamin supplement? And for my husband?

____

____

Do we need to change our diets in any way? (*in other words, we currently follow Atkins, Zone, Vegan, Lactose Intolerant, Blood Type, etc.*)

Do we need to stop taking any prescribed medications?

Anti-Acids	Appetite Suppressants	Hemorrhoid Treatments
Anti-Anxiety	Birth Control	Indigestion
Antibiotics	Blood Pressure	Laxatives
Anti-Coagulants	Cancer	Nasal Sprays
Anti-Depressants	Cholesterol	Pain
Anti-Gas	Cold	Seizure
Anti-Inflammatory	Diuretics	Steroids
Anti-Itch Products	Fungal and/or Yeast Infections	Sedatives

Can we continue taking over-the-counter medications? *(refer to "prescribed medications" checklist on previous page)*

Can we continue taking herbal products? *(bring a list of all herbal products that you currently use)*

I was adopted ☐ yes ☐ no.

My husband was adopted ☐ yes ☐ no.

Will my work environment (explain)… our home environment (explain)… or my hobbies (explain) harm my chances of conceiving and/or having a healthy baby? *(bring a list of all substances with which you come into contact, or inhale)*

Will my husband's work environment (explain)… or his hobbies (explain) harm my chances of conceiving and/or having a healthy baby? *(bring a list of all substances with which your husband comes into contact, or inhales)*

My blood type is ________.

My husband's blood type is ________.

I have had a Blood Transfusion ☐ yes ☐ no.

Date(s) ____________________________

Explain ____________________________

Should I be concerned about toxoplasmosis?

I have a history of problems with anesthesia ☐ yes ☐ no.

Explain ____________________________

VACCINATIONS YOU MAY NEED

If possible, bring your vaccination record or history:

- Chicken Pox
- Hepatitis A
- Hepatitis B
- HIB (Haemophilus Influenza Type B)
- Measles
- Mumps
- PCV (Pneumococcal Conjugate Vaccine)
- Polio
- Rubella

Should I receive a "flu shot" against influenza?

Should I receive a Chicken Pox vaccination?

Should I receive a vaccination to prevent Hepatitis B?

Should I receive a Lyme Disease vaccination, if available?

Should I receive a Tetanus Booster?

TESTING THAT COULD BE DONE

Should I be tested for Cystic Fibrosis?

Should my husband be tested for Cystic Fibrosis?

Should I be tested for Cytomegalovirus?

Should I be tested for Fifth Disease?

Should I be tested for Fragile "X" Syndrome?

Should I be tested for Group B Strep?

Should I be tested for Tuberculosis?

My ethnic background is ______________________________.

My husband's ethnic background is ________________________.

If you are of Eastern European Jewish decent: Should I receive a Tay-Sachs Disease blood test?

If you are of African American decent: Should I receive a Sickle Cell Disease blood test?

If you are of African American or Southern Asian decent: Should I receive a Thalassemia blood test?

If you are 35 years old or older… or if there is a family history: Should I receive genetic screening and counseling to discuss chromosomal defects such as Down Syndrome?

YOUR PERSONAL MEDICAL HISTORIES

☐ you **ABORTIONS**

☐ you **ANOVULATION**

☐ you **DIETHYLSTILBESTROL** (DES)

☐ you **ENDOMETRIOSIS**

☐ you **OVARIAN CYST**

☐ you **PELVIC INFLAMMATORY DISEASE (PID)**

☐ you **POLYCYSTIC OVARIAN SYNDROME (PCO)**

☐ you ☐ him **ACNE**

☐ you ☐ him **ALLERGIES**

☐ you ☐ him **ANEMIA**

☐ you ☐ him **ASTHMA**

☐ you ☐ him **CANCER**

☐ you ☐ him **CYSTIC FIBROSIS**

☐ you ☐ him **DIABETES**

☐ you ☐ him **DIGESTIVE PROBLEMS**

☐ you ☐ him **EATING DISORDERS** (Anorexia, Bulimia)

☐ you ☐ him **EPILEPSY**

☐ you ☐ him **FRAGILE "X" SYNDROME**

☐ you ☐ him **GENITAL WARTS**

☐ you ☐ him **GONORRHEA/CHLAMYDIA**

- [ ] you [ ] him **HEPATITIS A, B, C**
- [ ] you [ ] him **HERPES**
- [ ] you [ ] him **HIGH BLOOD PRESSURE**
- [ ] you [ ] him **HIV/AIDS**
- [ ] you [ ] him **HYPERTENSION**
- [ ] you [ ] him **KIDNEY DISEASE**
- [ ] you [ ] him **LIVER DISEASE**
- [ ] you [ ] him **LUPUS**
- [ ] you [ ] him **MENTAL ILLNESS**
- [ ] you [ ] him **MIGRAINES**
- [ ] you [ ] him **OVULATION/HORMONAL DISORDERS**
- [ ] you [ ] him **PHENYLKETONURIA (PKU)**
- [ ] you [ ] him **RHEUMATOID ARTHRITIS**
- [ ] you [ ] him **SEIZURES**
- [ ] you [ ] him **SURGERIES/CHEMOTHERAPY/RADIATION**
- [ ] you [ ] him **SYPHILIS**
- [ ] you [ ] him **THYROID DISEASE**

☐ you ☐ him **URINARY TRACT INFECTIONS**

☐ you ☐ him **YEAST INFECTIONS**

Other(s)

____

____

____

____

YOUR FAMILY MEDICAL HISTORIES

Be aware if there is a **Family History** (maternal & paternal) of the following, in either **YOUR FAMILY** or **HIS FAMILY**:

☐ your family ☐ his family **ADDICTIONS**

Explain: ______________________________

☐ your ☐ his **ANEMIA**

Explain: ______________________________

☐ your ☐ his **ASTHMA, TUBERCULOSIS,** or any lung disease

Explain: ______________________________

☐ your ☐ his **CANCER** (cervical, breast, prostate, testicular)
Explain: ______________________________

☐ your ☐ his **CARDIAC/NEURAL TUBE DEFECTS**

Explain: ______________________________

☐ your ☐ his **CEREBRAL PALSY**

Explain: ____

☐ your ☐ his **CLEFT LIP/PALATE**

Explain: ____

☐ your ☐ his **CONGENITAL ADRENAL HYPERPLASIA**

Explain: ____

☐ your ☐ his **CROHN'S DISEASE**

Explain: ____

☐ your ☐ his **CYSTIC FIBROSIS**

Explain: ____

☐ your ☐ his **DIABETES**

Explain: ____

☐ your ☐ his **DIETHYLSTILBESTROL (DES)**
(my mother took in 19__)

Explain: ____

☐ your ☐ his **DIGESTIVE PROBLEMS**

Explain: ____

☐ your family ☐ his family **DOWN SYNDROME/MENTAL RETARDATION**

Explain: ______________________________

☐ your ☐ his **EPILEPSY**

Explain: ______________________________

☐ your ☐ his **HEART DISEASE**

Explain: ______________________________

☐ your ☐ his **HEMOPHILIA A/BLEEDING DISORDERS**

Explain: ______________________________

☐ your ☐ his **HEPATITIS/LIVER DISEASES**

Explain: ______________________________

☐ your ☐ his **HIGH BLOOD PRESSURE**

Explain: ______________________________

☐ your ☐ his **HUNTINGTON'S DISEASE**

Explain: ______________________________

☐ your ☐ his **KIDNEY DISEASE**

Explain: ______________________________

☐ your ☐ his **LUPUS**

Explain: ______________________________

☐ your ☐ his **MENTAL ILLNESS**

Explain: ______________________________

☐ your ☐ his **MENTAL RETARDATION**

Explain: ______________________________

☐ your ☐ his **MIGRAINES**

Explain: ______________________________

☐ your ☐ his **MISCARRIAGE**

Explain: ______________________________

☐ your ☐ his **MULTIPLE BIRTHS**

Explain: ______________________________

☐ your ☐ his **MUSCULAR DYSTROPHY**

Explain: ______________________________

☐ your ☐ his **PHENYLKETONURIA (PKU)**

Explain: ______________________________

☐ your family ☐ his family **POLYCYSTIC KIDNEY DISEASE**

Explain: ____________________

☐ your ☐ his **PREMATURE OVARIAN FAILURE** (cessation of menstruation before the age of 40) -

Explain: ____________________

☐ your ☐ his **SICKLE CELL ANEMIA**

Explain: ____________________

☐ your ☐ his **SPINA BIFIDA/SPINE DEFECTS**

Explain: ____________________

☐ your ☐ his **TAY-SACHS DISEASE**

Explain: ____________________

☐ your ☐ his **THALASSEMIA**

Explain: ____________________

☐ your ☐ his **THYROID DISEASE**

Explain: ____________________

☐ your ☐ his **VASO VAGAL REACTION**

Explain: ____________________

Other(s) explain:

☐ your ☐ his ________________________________

☐ your ☐ his ________________________________

☐ your ☐ his ________________________________

☐ your ☐ his ________________________________

☐ your ☐ his ________________________________

☐ your ☐ his ________________________________

☐ your ☐ his ________________________________

☐ your ☐ his ________________________________

☐ your ☐ his ________________________________

☐ your ☐ his ________________________________

☐ your ☐ his ________________________________

☐ your ☐ his ________________________________

☐ your ☐ his ________________________________

Index

A

B

C

G

H

L

M

PQ

S

U

V

W

XYZ

ACKNOWLEDGMENTS

Grateful acknowledgement is made to the following for permission to print the material, or copyrighted material, listed below:

J. Francois Eid, M.D., www.urologicalcare.com: Used by permission of J. Francois Eid, M.D., Center for Urological Care, 50 East 69th Street, New York, NY 10021.

Alan Hirsch, M.D., Neurological Director, Smell + Taste Treatment and Research Foundation, Chicago, IL: Used by permission of Dr. Alan Hirsch, www.smellandtaste.org.

Excerpts from THE GODDESS' GUIDE TO LOVE, Copyright © 1999 by Margie Lapanja, with permission of Conari Press, an imprint of Red Wheel/Weiser, Boston, MA and York Beach, ME. To order call: 1-800-423-7087.

THE GOOD SPELL BOOK by Gillian Kemp: Copyright © 1999 by Gillian Kemp. Used by permission of Little, Brown and Company, (Inc): Excerpts from pp. 39-41, 73, 74, 100, 102, 105, 112.

Journal of The Royal Society of Medicine, Anthony M. Perks & Bailey, D.M., *Stonehenge: a view from medicine*: Used by permission of Journal of The Royal Society of Medicine, 1 Wimpole Street, London W1G 0AE.

WISE WOMAN HERBAL FOR THE CHILDBEARING YEAR by Susun S. Weed: 1985-2004 by Susun S. Weed. Used by permission of Susun S. Weed at Ash Tree Publishing, P.O. Box 64, Woodstock, NY 12498.

www.elevatedconceptions.com: Copyright © 2004 ONEUP INNOVATIONS, LLC / Copyright © 2004 just pillows, inc. Used by permission of Deb Burak, President, just pillows, inc.

www.motherisk.org: Motherisk Program, The Hospital for Sick Children, Toronto, Canada. Used by permission of Dr. G. Koren, M.D., FRCPC.

www.rabbitsfootmeadery.com: Rabbits Foot Meadery, 1122 Aster Avenue, Suite J, Sunnyvale, CA 94086. Used by permission of www.rabbitsfootmeadery.com.

REFERENCES

Albertson, Ellen and Michael. *Temptations*. New York: Simon & Schuster, 2002.

Biziou, Barbara. *The Joy of Rituals*. New York: Golden Books, 1999.

Botkin, B. A. *A Treasury of American Folklore*. New York: Crown Publishers, 1944.

__________. *Bride's Little Book of Customs and Keepsakes*. New York: Crown Publishing, 1994.

Cooper, J.C. *An Illustrated Encyclopaedia of Traditional Symbols*. New York: Thames and Hudson, 1999.

Campbell, Joseph. *The Hero With A Thousand Faces*. New York: MJF Books, 1949.

Cunningham, Scott. *Encyclopedia of Magical Herbs*. St. Paul, MN: Llewellyn Publications, 2002.

England, Allison. *Aromatherapy and Massage for Mother and Baby*. Rochester, VT: Healing Arts Press, 2000.

Gawain, Shakti. *Creative Visualization*. Novato, CA: Nataraj Publishing, 2002.

Keville, Kathy. *Herbs for Health and Healing*. Emmaus, PA: Rodale Press, 1996.

__________. *Language of Flowers*. New York: Lorenz Books, 1997.

McQuillar, Tayannah. *Rootwork – Using the Folk Magick of Black America for Love, Success and Money*. New York: Fireside, 2003.

Melody. *Love Is In The Earth – A Kaleidoscope of Crystals*. Wheat Ridge, CO: Earth-Love Publishing House, 2002.

Miller, Manya DeLeon. *The Complete Fertility Organizer: A Guidebook and Record Keeper for Women*. New York: John Wiley & Sons, Inc. 1999.

Mindell, Earl. *Earl Mindell's New Herb Bible*. New York: Fireside, 2000.

McIntyre, Anne. *Drink To Your Health*. New York: Simon & Schuster, 2000.

Needleman, Jacob. *A Little Book On Love*. New York: Dell Publishing, 1996.

Ohlig, Adelheid. *Luna Yoga – Vital Fertility and Sexuality*. Woodstock, NY: Ash Tree Publishing, 1994.

Parvati, Jeannine B., Baker, Frederick, and Slayton, Tamara. *Conscious Conception*. Sevier, UT: Freestone Publishing, 1986.

Telesco, Patricia. *Goddess In My Pocket*. San Francisco: HarperCollins, 1998.

Waters, Frank. *Book Of The Hopi*. New York: Ballantine Books, 1969.

Teish, Luisah. *Jump Up – Good Times throughout the Seasons with Celebrations From Around the World*. Berkeley, CA: Conari Press, 2000.

Williams, Phyllis S. *Nourishing Your Unborn Child*. New York: Avon Books, 1974.

Waldherr, Kris. *Sacred Animals*. New York: HarperCollins, 2001.

Order Form

QUICK ORDER FORM

FAX ORDERS: 401-253-1832. Fax a copy of this form.

WEB ORDERS: www.pinksandblues.com

POSTAL ORDERS:
Pinks and Blues Publishing
P.O. Box 687
Bristol, RI 02809

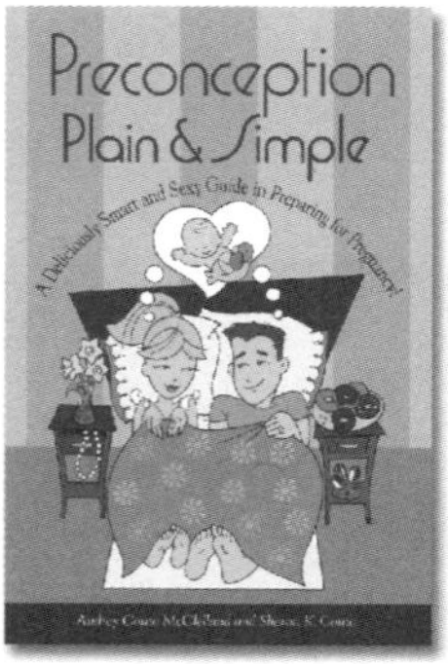

Please send the following book:

Preconception Plain & Simple

Name ______________________________

Address ______________________________

City ______________ State ________ Zip ________

Telephone ______________________________

Email Address ______________________________

SHIPPING / HANDLING
USA: $4.00 for first book and $2.00 for each additional book.
International: $9.00 for first book and $5.00 for each additional book.

Book(s) ___	@$19.95ea =	______
Shipping	+	______
Tax*	+	______
TOTAL	=	______

*Orders shipped to RI and CT, add 7%; MA, add 5%.

Payment: ☐ Check (payable to: **Pinks and Blues Publishing**)
or Credit Card: ☐ Visa ☐ MasterCard

Name on Card ______________________________

Card Number ______________________ Exp. Date ________